Straight Talk *about* Breast Cancer

From Diagnosis to Recovery

A Guide for the Entire Family

Suzanne W. Braddock, M.D.
John J. Edney, M.D.
Jane M. Kercher, M.D.
Melanie Morrissey Clark

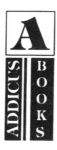

Omaha, Nebraska

An Addicus Nonfiction Book

Addicus Books
P.O. Box 45327
Omaha, Neb., 68145
Web site: www.AddicusBooks.com

ISBN# 1-886039-21-6

Cover design and illustrations by Jeff Reiner
Photography by Larry S. Ferguson

This book is not intended to serve as a substitute for a physician, nor do the authors intend to give medical advice contrary to an attending physician's.

Library of Congress Cataloging-in-Publication Data

   Straight talk about breast cancer : from diagnosis to recovery : a guide for the entire family / by Suzanne W. Braddock ... [et al.] . -- 1st ed.
      p.   cm.
   Includes bibliographical references.
   ISBN 1-886039-21-6 (trade paper)
   1. Breast--Cancer—Popular works. I. Braddock, Suzanne W. , 1942-
RC280 .B8 S75 1994
616 . 99'449--dc20

94-37848
CIP

Printed in the United States of America
10 9 8

Wind

I sit silent in the cold room, reading
when softly, a stir outside calls me away. It is the wind,
moving the frozen oaks and evergreens, pushing the
snow across the ice on the lake.
It is a sound both great and small,
the breath of God over the land
the voice of creation
giving life to this cold, barren landscape,
to my days of terror.
I feel the power embraced in that sound, and joy in the force that is greater than I,
greater than cancer, greater than all the pain in all the women.

- Suzanne W. Braddock, 1993

To all women diagnosed with breast cancer and their families.

Proceeds from this book will go toward helping
women with breast cancer obtain needed services.

Contents

Preface

Please read this book imagining that a very good friend is sitting close to you, giving you this introduction to the rest of your life with love and understanding.

Imagine your friend - who has indeed walked in your shoes - taking you by the hand and guiding you through the next few weeks.

Your friend wants to help you understand what is happening, and help you cope with the decisions and treatments ahead. She also wants to help your family and friends, for they are suffering with you.

Know there will come a time when you will go entire minutes without thinking of breast cancer - then hours, and even days. Of course, your life will never be the same. In fact, it will probably be *better* in many ways you would not have chosen, but will be delighted to discover.

The authors of this book reach out to you as dear friends and offer you the hope of a complete recovery, along with the certainty that the journey from here will be one of growth, challenge and change. That is, after all, what life is about.

BY SUZANNE W. BRADDOCK, M.D.
DIAGNOSED WITH BREAST CANCER IN 1992

Introduction

Someone you know, someone you love, will get breast cancer.

Your friend, your aunt, your mother, your daughter, yourself. The fact is, if you are an American woman, you are at risk. One in eight of us - should we all live to age 85 - will get breast cancer. About 1,400 American men developed the disease in 1996.

How do we deal with this epidemic? How does each woman handle this intensely personal crisis?

The rest of my life started April 1, 1992, with a phone call from my friend and colleague, informing me that my outpatient biopsy had been diagnosed malignant. I reacted, as do most women, with the usual irrational certainty that I was going to die, and soon. I was 49.

Breast cancer strikes enough women to fill a 747 aircraft every day. Every third day, one of those planes crashes and kills all on board. The good news is, most women survive breast cancer. And not just five-year, disease-free survival, either. Real, long-lasting, bounce-the-grandkids-on-your-knee survival.

Although a physician, I am a dermatologist and knew little more about breast cancer other than what I had learned in medical school in the late 1970s. I had assisted several patients who had died from the disease, and knew I didn't want to get it. So I dutifully saw my physician every year for an exam (*right*), had a baseline mammogram between ages 35 and 40 (*right*), had a mammogram every other year between 40 and 50 (*right*), began scheduling annual mammograms when I was about to turn 50 (*right*) and practiced breast-self examinations on a regularly sporadic basis (*wrong*). As is true of many women, my breasts were "lumpy," making self-examination difficult to interpret. I relied on my physician and mammograms to keep me safe (*very wrong*). Today yearly mammograms are recommended after age 40.

Although most breast cancers strike women over age 50, a significant percentage show up in younger women. Many, but not all, of these young women are at high risk for developing the disease because they have the breast cancer gene in their families. But these women comprise between only 5 and 10 percent of the total breast cancer population.

Most women who develop breast cancer are not high risk. This is a fact many doctors and most patients fail to realize. To make matters worse, diagnosis in younger women is made more difficult because between 10 and 20 percent of their mammograms are false-negative: Cancer is present but the mammogram is unable to detect it due to the dense tissue in young breasts. By the time a tumor has become large enough to be felt, it has become large enough to significantly increase the risk of death.

Fortunately for me, not every malignancy "reads" the textbooks. Although my tumor was 2.2 centimeters - a little smaller than one inch - it had not yet spread to the lymph nodes when diagnosed, at least as far as current technology could determine.

I was disappointed that three doctors had examined me many times and failed to recommend a biopsy. I was disheartened that the mammogram had failed to detect such a mass. But I was most of all amazed that I had been so cavalier with the very things that could have diagnosed my tumor sooner: regular, monthly breast self-exams and insistence on a biopsy. Denial is a powerful thing.

Delay of diagnosis of breast cancer is a real problem in the younger woman. She is often told "it's just a cyst, we'll watch it" or "it's just a blocked milk duct - wait until you stop nursing." Many physicians have a real reluctance to tell a young woman she may have breast cancer. Nearly 75 percent of malpractice dollars deal with delay of breast cancer diagnosis.

What causes breast cancer? If only 5 percent of breast cancer patients are genetically predisposed to develop the disease, what about the rest of us? Most experts believe female hormones, in particular estrogen, play a significant role in the development or growth of breast cancer. Estrogen-like activity of various pesticides, such as DDT, has been linked with increased risk of breast cancer.

Women who, like myself, never gave birth are at increased risk, presumably because of increased ovulatory cycles and exposure to estrogen. In rare cases, pregnancy hormones can stimulate growth of a tumor already present but too small to detect. Early childbirth and breast-feeding seem to decrease the risk, possibly by limiting the amount of estrogen the body is exposed to over a lifetime. Even foods, such as broccoli, linked to decreased risk of cancer, may act at least in part by metabolizing estrogen to a less harmful form.

Obesity may increase the risk of breast cancer - but it has been shown to do so only in the postmenopausal woman. Dietary fat may act as a reservoir for pesticides, and limiting fat intake has been shown in some studies to prevent both the onset of cancer and the spread of known cancer. Other studies have failed to confirm these findings.

Most premenopausal women have tumors that are estrogen-receptor negative, however. These tumors are thought to be less dependent upon that hormone for growth, and less responsive to certain hormonal therapies. Other factors make premenopausal cancers more dangerous, including faster-growing and dividing cells, cells that have atypical amounts of DNA, and many other factors still actively being researched. Many tumors - like mine - possess a mixture of features that make predicting their future behavior difficult at best.

Your immediate future, however, is certain. You may be facing weeks or months of therapy, disruption of your normal routine, adjustment to new fears and fatigue. But what you fear most - death from breast cancer - may or may not occur. Even if the worst happens, it may be years down the road. By that time, new methods of cancer treatment will be available. In the meantime, you may come to see your struggle with cancer diagnosis as a gift - a precious signpost showing you that the real value and meaning of life lies in the little moments, the daily rituals of love given and received. Does not the real value of life lie in its quality rather than its length? Cancer survivors everywhere speak often of their cancer as the best thing that has happened to them, allowing them to place importance on the things that last.

Since 1988, breast cancer patients have been uniformly offered chemotherapy if their tumors were of a certain size or in a high-risk category for future recurrence. Disease-free survival - perhaps even overall survival - can be increased by giving this "adjuvant chemotherapy." It has been a real growth industry for the wig makers.

The usual chemotherapy for early stage breast cancer, while no picnic, is definitely do-able. Most women fear chemo not only for hair loss, but for nausea. Luckily, newer drugs help eliminate the violent retching Hollywood features in those chemo movies. Other drugs help the bone marrow make more cells, preventing delays in treatment.

So your bad hair day extends to about nine months, and you are a bit nauseated and fatigued. My daughter, Gail, had a lot of fun playing with my wig - or as we called it, "the muskrat."

Actually, I learned to like the ease with which I could wash my "hair" - swish it in a bowl of suds, rinse and hang to dry. The possibilities were endless - snatching it off on the hot drive home from work and chuckling at the startled expressions on the faces of other drivers.

Going through surgery and chemotherapy mobilizes you, and it is easy to focus on the one-third done, then halfway through, then done. Your eyelashes return, and before you know it, you're ready to donate your wig to the American Cancer Society's wig bank. Then you climb the hill behind your house without gasping for breath and, finally, go an entire day without thinking about breast cancer.

My days now, after chemotherapy, are as precious in their possible brevity as the glimpse of a small garden behind a city brownstone. These are the good days. They have shown me, in a poignant and powerful way, that life is best lived by us all, diagnosed with cancer or not, in a state of radical trust. Trust and trust and trust some more. None of us knows the limits of our days, but we do know Who limits them. And that is all we need to know.

CHAPTER ONE

Diagnosis

The words "breast cancer" make every woman uneasy. To the woman first diagnosed with the disease, they are devastating.

Yet viewed from a different perspective, diagnosis is the first step toward treatment and survival. In actuality, breast cancer diagnosis saves lives.

Breast lumps are discovered in one of three ways: by the woman herself, by a doctor during a physical examination, or by a mammogram.

Although about 80 percent of breast lumps are benign, early detection of a malignant lump can dramatically increase survival.

Early detection means the cancer is small when it is detected - usually no larger than 2 centimeters (a little less than one inch) - and has not spread to the lymph nodes

"At the time of diagnosis, I was so frightened. I thought for sure I was going to die in a month or two. Breast cancer had always been my greatest fear.

"My husband and children surrounded me with love, which was the best thing they could have done. They were always considerate, but not pampering.

"Instead of dwelling on 'Why me?' my motto became, 'Why not me?'"

-Carolyn, age 65

around the breast.

Breast Self-Examination

Because more than 75 percent of malignant lumps are found by the woman herself, medical professionals encourage women to make breast self-examination (BSE) part of their monthly routine.

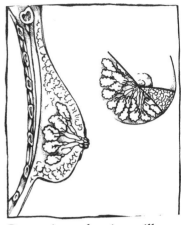

Breast tissue showing milk ducts and lobules.

Women should start monthly examinations as soon as their breasts develop, or at the latest by age 20. Because the breasts tend to become firmer and fuller a few days prior to the menstrual period, pre-menopausal women should perform BSE about 10 days after the beginning of their periods. Post-menopausal women should examine their breasts on the same day every month.

Women who are afraid to practice self-examination must realize that finding a small tumor is much better than finding a large one. Even if you have lumpy breasts and are unsure of what to look for, regularly examining your breasts will help you recognize any changes.

It is never safe to stop doing BSE. Women should practice it all their lives.

Women who have had breast surgery also should perform BSE on a regular basis. If you've had a mastectomy, examine the incision for firmness or discoloration and search for lumps above the collarbone and in the armpit. Practicing BSE on the opposite breast also is extremely important.

Women who have had breast cancer sometimes feel they are immune to developing a second malignancy in the other breast. This is not the case. In fact, the risk can be quite high with certain types of breast cancer. Discuss your risk and any changes you detect with your doctor.

How To Do BSE

1. Stand before a mirror. Inspect your breasts for anything unusual, such as any discharge from the nipple, or a puckering, dimpling or scaling of the skin. If you've had a mastectomy, inspect the scar for new swelling, lumps, redness or color change.

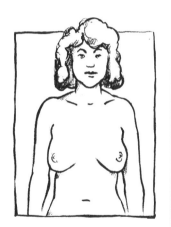

2. Watching closely in the mirror, clasp your hands behind your head and press your hands forward. Next, press your hands firmly on your hips and bow

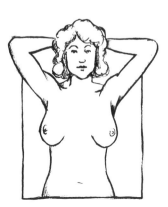

"When I told Gary that I had to have a biopsy, he remained at my side through it all. My husband took over making decisions that I never realized he could before my diagnosis."

-Fran, age 47

An estimated 184,300 new invasive cases among women were diagnosed in the United States during 1996. About 1,400 new cases of breast cancer were diagnosed in men the same year. Incidence rates have increased about 4 percent a year in the past but have recently begun to level off.

Questions to ask your doctor regarding your biopsy:

•What type of biopsy will I have?

•Will the entire lump be removed, or just part of it?

•Does the procedure require general or local anesthesia?

• How long will the biopsy take?

•Can the biopsy be performed on an outpatient basis?

•When will I know the results from the pathology report?

•If I do have cancer, how much time will I have to research my treatment options?

•What studies will be performed on my biopsy?

slightly toward the mirror as you pull your shoulders and elbows forward.

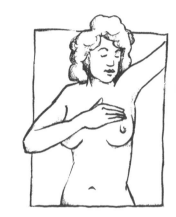

3. Raise your right arm. Using three or four fingers of your other hand, explore your breast firmly, carefully and thoroughly.

Beginning at the outer edge, press the flat part of your fingers in small circles, moving the circles slowly around the breast. Gradually work toward the nipple. Be sure to cover the entire breast. Pay special attention to the area between the breast and underarm, including the underarm itself. Feel for any unusual lump or mass under the skin.

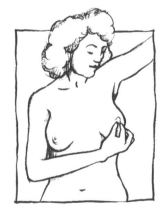

4. Gently squeeze the nipple and look for a discharge. Raise your left arm and repeat Step 3. Lumps, thickening and puckering of the skin are changes you should bring to your doctor's attention.

5. Repeat steps three and four lying down. Lie flat on your back, raise your right arm over

your head and place a pillow or folded towel under your shoulder. This position flattens the breast and makes it easier to examine. Use the same circular motion described earlier. Repeat on the other side.

Mammography

Mammography, the best screening process currently available for breast cancer, is used not only to search for lumps but also to look at them after they have been found. In other words, the second step after a woman or her doctor finds a lump is mammography.

A mammogram is an x-ray which pictures the tissues of the breast. It is performed by a radiologist or an x-ray technician under the supervision of a radiologist.

Women also should have mammograms at these times:

•Once between ages 35 and 40, to establish a picture of the breasts against which future conditions can be measured.

•The Journal of the American Medical Association recommends yearly mammograms for women ages 40 and older (old recommendations were every one to two years in ages 40 to 50). About 29,000 cases of breast cancer are diagnosed in women between ages 40 and 50 each year, while 33,000 cases are diagnosed in women ages 50 to 60. Because the number of breast cancer cases is nearly equivalent in both age groups, it makes sense to have annual mammograms beginning at age 40. Tumors in young

> "My doctor found it in a routine mammogram shortly after I turned 40. They told me it was positive. I immediately started to cry, and thought I was going to die. As you can see, I didn't."
>
> *-Alice, age 46*

> Approximately 1 in 2,000 pregnant or lactating women has breast cancer, and 1 to 2 percent of breast cancers are diagnosed in pregnant women.

"I was 32 when I felt a lump in my left breast and went to my family physician. A mammogram showed no abnormalities. Thank God the general surgeon was very cautious and asked me if I'd like to have the lump removed just to be safe. Cancer did not run in my family, so I had no inkling that I would have it.

"That lump was benign, but he happened to dig down deeper and found a malignant tumor against my chest wall. So it's a miracle that I found this benign lump, because otherwise I would never have had a mammogram until I was 35 or 40, and I never would have had a breast biopsy. It was a fluke that I think probably saved my life."

-Dianna, age 32

women grow quickly. Annual mammograms could diagnose tumors early enough to save lives.

- Every year after age 40.
- Annually if she has had any type of breast cancer, no matter what her age.
- If she has had a sister or mother diagnosed with breast cancer, she should have mammograms beginning 10 years earlier than the age at which her family member was diagnosed.

Abnormal results of a mammogram include a group of small, white dots (**clustered microcalcifications**) and a star-shaped (**spiculated**) suspicious mass or nodule. **Benign** (non-cancerous) tumors or cysts appear to have smooth, clear margins. Another test, called an ultrasound, uses sound waves to detect whether a mass is solid, or cystic and filled with fluid. A cyst would create a dark shadow on the ultrasound image.

Although not widely used, a new test, Miraluma, can visualize the increased blood vessels in and around breast tumors. This test is particularly useful when the mammogram fails to visualize a lump — especially in young women whose breasts are dense. The test is very sensitive and specific.

Positron Emission Tomography (PET) and Magnetic Resonance Imaging (MRI) scanning are other techniques available in certain areas of the country. Both techniques are being used as diagnostic tools before biopsy. MRI and Miraluma are being evaluated for detecting early recurrences in women who have had lumpectomies.

Biopsy

A biopsy removes tissue from the suspicious area so it can be examined under a microscope by a pathologist. Most breast biopsies reveal no malignancy. Eighty percent reveal benign breast conditions.

A suspicious lump does not always show up on a mammogram. And whether or not it does, a medical professional most likely will recommend a biopsy if he or she can feel it.

A persistent lump should always be biopsied, regardless of family history or the presence or absence of other risk factors. Although some doctors try to diagnose a lump by examination alone, the only certain way to establish a lump's nature is by biopsy. Women should insist on one.

Needle Aspiration

Fine-needle aspiration, one of several kinds of biopsies, serves as both diagnosis and treatment for a non-malignant cyst. During needle aspiration, a fine, hollow needle is inserted into the lump under local anesthesia, and any fluid present is drawn into a syringe.

If fine-needle aspiration reveals a solid mass, the sample can be sent to a pathologist for analysis. But even if the

> **"I always tried not to take this diagnosis and therapy too seriously. I often treated things lightly so the people around me would not be embarrassed or sad. For example, I often joked about how nice it would be not to have to wear a bra anymore."**
>
> *-Nancy, age 51*

> "When my mom first told me about her cancer, I was worried, like, 'Who's going to take care of me?' or 'What if she dies?' She was totally honest with me. I felt reassured because it wasn't like cancer was this deadly, mysterious thing that snuck up on someone."
>
> -Gail, age 13

pathologist's report comes back negative, meaning no cancer cells are seen, an open biopsy may still be recommended, because the needle occasionally misses cancer cells.

Next, a surgeon may opt for a core-needle biopsy. First, a small incision is made in the skin, and the large-caliber needle then removes a small wedge of tissue.

Again, if no malignant cells are found, the results are inconclusive and another biopsy may be performed. If, however, the second biopsy reveals cancer is present, the results are reliable.

Stereotactic Biopsy

Another method of obtaining tissue, stereotactic biopsy combines mammography and computer-directed needle placement to evaluate an abnormality the mammogram can see but the doctor can't feel. This procedure is performed with local anesthesia and takes between 30 and 90 minutes. Most women experience little discomfort as a result of stereotactic biopsy.

Formal or "Open" Biopsy

The two types of open biopsies are incisional and excisional. An incisional biopsy is performed if the tumor is large, and only a small piece of tissue is removed for examination. An excisional biopsy means the tumor is small and is removed completely. Open biopsies can be done on an

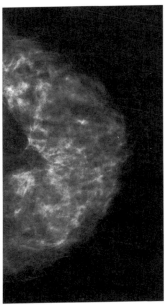

A normal mammogram.

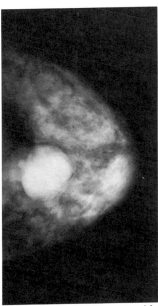

Mammogram showing cysts with smooth edges.

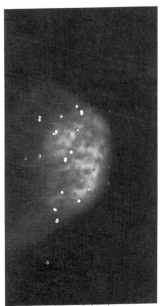

Mammogram with benign calcifications scattered throughout.

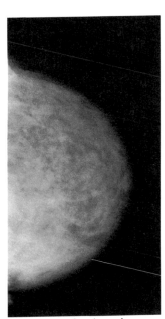

Mammogram showing a dense pattern - usually seen in younger women.

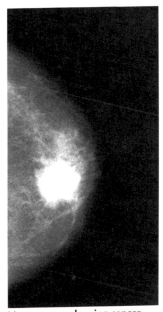

Mammogram showing cancer. Note irregular edges.

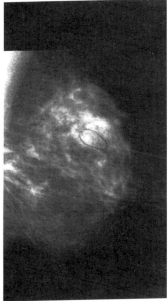

Mammogram with a group of clustered microcalcifications

"Shortly after my diagnosis, a co-worker came running up to me as I was getting off the elevator at work with outstretched arms and said, 'You poor thing. What are you going to do?' I gave her my bitchy look and told her I was fine and I would do what I needed to do.

"That's one thing about menopause - I can always mention it in my apology."
-Roxanne, age 52

outpatient basis. A pathologist examines the removed tissue under a microscope, looking for the following:

1. How large is the tumor?

Tumors are grouped according to size, because size - along with other factors - determines treatment. In general, small tumors are less than two centimeters (less than one inch). Tumors between two and five centimeters (up to two inches) make up the next category, and tumors more than five centimeters (two inches) are considered large.

2. Do the blood vessels or lymph vessels contain cancer cells?

If the answer is yes, a woman is more likely to be advised to undergo additional treatment, such as chemotherapy and/or radiation therapy, to prevent tumor spread.

3. Is the tumor well-differentiated or poorly differentiated?

Well-differentiated cells look more like normal breast cells. Poorly differentiated cells indicate a more aggressive tumor.

4. Is the tumor diploid?

Diploid tumor cells contain normal amounts of DNA, resembling normal breast cells, and have a favorable prognosis. **Aneuploid tumor cells** have abnormal amounts of DNA, a less-favorable prognosis and are more aggressive.

5. S-Phase: How fast are the cells reproducing?

This test simply measures the percentage of cells that are dividing in the tumor. The typical range is from 1 to 25 percent. Interpretation of results varies with tumor type and from lab to lab.

6. Does the tumor have estrogen and/or progesterone receptors?

Even very small tissue samples can be tested for receptors for the female hormones estrogen and progesterone. Receptors are areas on a cell's surface which resemble a "lock." A hormone fits that area like a "key." Cell functions are thought to be affected when the "key" is inserted.

Some tumor cells show a high number of receptors for these hormones. Because estrogen and progesterone circulating in the blood may stimulate tumor growth, doctors use this finding to make important treatment decisions, such as the use of anti-hormone medications.

Tumors with a high percentage of cells positive for estrogen and/or progesterone receptors usually have a favorable prognosis. Post-menopausal women often have a high percentage of cells positive for estrogen and progesterone receptors. This usually is seen with well-differentiated, slow-growing tumors, but exceptions occur.

About two-thirds of premenopausal women have estro-

> **"Telling my children was so difficult that I just didn't. I guess I didn't want them to worry or come rushing home when they couldn't afford it. They still don't know I had the surgery."**
>
> *-Linda, age 44*

"The tumor was not found on my first mammogram, and my doctor believed I was feeling an overworked muscle. I continued on for three years, believing this, until I noticed a decrease in breast size. At this time, another mammogram was done, and a biopsy advised. The tumor was five centimeters, but I thanked God that it had not metastasized.

"My advice to women is to know your body and perform monthly breast self-exams. See your doctor if you have any concerns, and if you have any doubts, get a second opinion."

-Dianna, age 47

gen-receptor-negative tumors. This is thought to increase the risk of mortality by 5 percent. Physicians often recommend more aggressive chemotherapeutic regimens when a tumor is estrogen-negative.

Biopsy Results

Although a pathologist can obtain preliminary results by looking at a "frozen section" while the patient is in the operating room, this method is not always accurate, and it generally takes one or two days to obtain the results of a "permanent section" biopsy. The permanent section is the most accurate method.

Types of Breast Cancer

The two most common types of breast cancer are:

1. **Ductal** (starts in the milk ducts)

   a. **in situ** (has not spread through the wall of the milk duct, where it originated. This is technically a precancerous condition); or

   b. **invasive** (has spread through the wall of the milk duct, into the surrounding breast tissue).

2. **Lobular carcinoma** (starts in the milk lobules)

   a. in situ; or

   b. invasive.

Lobular carcinoma has a high risk of being present in both breasts.

Other rare types of breast cancers exist, and carry a slightly different prognosis. Each rare type occurs less than 1 to 1.5 percent of the time.

One-Step Vs. Two-Step Procedure

Except in rare cases, the days of one-step biopsies and mastectomies have practically disappeared. The few who do opt for them make arrangements in advance with their surgeons. For example, a woman who already has had one mastectomy and discovers a suspicious lump in the opposite breast may arrange for a biopsy immediately followed by mastectomy.

For most women, a delay of one to two weeks between a biopsy and definitive surgery is common and considered safe. This two-step procedure gives women diagnosed with breast cancer time to research their treatment options. Some doctors schedule surgery during a particular phase of the menstrual cycle.

Pre-Operative Studies

Most physicians will order several tests before surgery to determine whether or not the cancer has spread to other organs. These include a chest x-ray, bone scan, liver ultrasound and/or scan, and blood tests.

> "I got myself through my initial anxiety regarding my diagnosis by saying to myself, 'Well, I'm alive today and I will live today to the hilt.' By fearing death, I figured I was dying all the time instead of living - it really only takes a little while to die, and I would live until then."
>
> *-Suzanne, age 50*

CHAPTER TWO

Coping

Most women, upon hearing the words "breast cancer," immediately think they're going to die.

Old memories of family members, friends or neighbors who suffered from cancer and quickly died contribute to this fear, which today often proves unfounded.

Thanks to medical advances which have dramatically lengthened the survival rates of most cancers, this much-feared disease is no longer equated with imminent death. While still a serious and life-threatening disease, breast cancer has become a treatable form of cancer, and women who develop it can and do live long lives.

Support In Stressful Times

Studies indicate that the diagnostic phase is an extremely stressful time for women with breast cancer, marked by high

"Sometimes all I needed was someone to sit and cry with or to offer a reassuring hug. But some people don't know what to do, and they unintentionally say the wrong things. For example, telling someone with cancer not to worry is like telling someone not to breathe. My own mother said to me, 'If you have to have cancer, this is the best kind to have.' I guess people just don't think."

-Marcia, age 44

> "I advise every woman diagnosed with breast cancer to join a support group. It's the best thing I ever did, and I've made some lifelong friends who truly understand what I've been through."
>
> *-Linda, age 47*

anxiety, uncertainty and difficulty in making decisions. However, some research suggests that women who are given a choice about the type of surgery they have experience less anxiety and depression before and after surgery than women who are not given a choice.

Most women experience the highest level of depression after surgery, when they return home from the hospital.

Experts say talking about the illness is important to a woman's well-being. While most women instinctively turn to significant others, close friends and relatives, they sometimes are surprised to find not everyone can provide the support needed.

Some friends and relatives - and even significant others - cope by avoiding the subject entirely. Others don't call or write at all. Still others come through with flying colors, sending cheerful cards and letters, visiting when appropriate and keeping in touch by telephone.

Support Groups

A woman's breast cancer also can bring treasured new friends, particularly if she joins a support group. One study revealed that women with metastatic breast cancer who participated regularly in a breast cancer support group lived an average of 18 months longer than those who didn't join a group. Support groups are made up of women of all ages and from all walks of life. Newcomers are warmly welcomed.

Most large hospitals offer support groups specifically for women with breast cancer. The women who take advantage of them report that the meetings give them strength. Hearing others express fears and share valuable information helps them realize they are not alone. Most women find great comfort in that knowledge.

Unfortunately, the women who could profit most from a support group - those who are depressed, anxious and fear the worst - often don't join one.

The National Coalition for Cancer Survivorship (NCCS) helps cancer survivors and their families start local support groups or contact existing ones. To find a local NCCS group, call the national office at 1-505-764-9956.

Meditation, Nutrition and Exercise

Women with breast cancer find taking time out to pamper or take special care of themselves improves their mental, as well as physical, well-being.

Meditating for 10 to 20 minutes twice a day promotes an overall sense of peace, and has been shown to help the body fight the damaging effects of stress. Some women like to meditate by silently repeating the word "peace," while calmly pushing away distractions in the mind. Another form of meditation - imagery - visualizes the body healing cancer cells.

Eating right makes many women feel they're doing

> "My husband and I had some of our best talks when we took our daily walks. It not only got us out of the house, it also gave us a chance to really talk in a nonconfrontational setting. We still take our walks today."
>
> -*Dianna, age 33*

What husbands can do to help their wives:

• Tell her you love her daily.
• Hug her daily.
• Fix meals when she's having radiation or chemotherapy treatment.
• Clean or have someone clean the house.
• Listen to her fears rather than simply reassuring her everything will be OK.
• Realize you don't need to be in control, you just need to be there for her.
• Tell her she's pretty.
• Do something nice for yourself.
• Take her for a walk and hold her hand.
• Check the refrigerator and get the milk, eggs and bread *before* they run out.
• Keep medical bills paid and avoid discussing them during her treatment.
• Try to take her out to dinner once a month.
• Set goals together.

something to fight the cancer. And they may well be. A low-fat diet has been shown to decrease risk of developing breast and other cancers.

Raw foods that may inhibit cancer growth include broccoli, cabbage, brussels sprouts, cauliflower, mustard greens, turnip greens, kale and radishes.

Animal studies have shown that dietary fiber also can reduce the risk of breast cancer, perhaps by influencing the body's metabolism of estrogen, which studies have implicated in promoting growth of breast malignancies.

Other studies suggest vitamins A and C and beta-carotene may protect against cancer. And more than 100 studies have shown significant decreases in cancer rates among people whose diets are high in the fruits and vegetables that contain these vitamins. Foods that contain beta-carotene include apricots, beet greens, black-eyed peas, cantaloupe, carrots, sweet potatoes, pumpkin and spinach.

Other foods thought to inhibit cancer include fresh garlic and soy products, such as tofu. Choose low-fat tofu, however, because the regular version is high in fat.

A low-fat diet goes hand-in-hand with exercise, which can improve both mental and physical health. Even 10 minutes of exercise twice a week benefits the heart and bones, especially for women past menopause. Natural killer cells, those which fight off tumor cells, increase in number after exercise.

Husbands and Significant Others

Breast cancer, like all cancers, is a disease that affects the entire family. Husbands and significant others experience intense emotions and fears when the women they love are diagnosed with and treated for breast cancer.

Because everyone copes and expresses emotions differently, there is no "right way" for men to react. The strong silent type may hesitate to discuss his feelings for fear of burdening his wife. Other men either completely ignore the disease or overcompensate by being excessively cheerful. Some men may find it difficult to talk about their fears because they aren't ready to face them.

Sometimes, women simply need to give their husbands permission to express their fears and feelings. Others find their husbands unable to provide needed support. These women seek out support from a friend, minister or counselor. There is nothing wrong with a husband who avoids talking about his wife's breast cancer. Everyone copes differently.

Lost In The Shuffle

The hospital phase is a particularly difficult time for spouses and significant others, who must juggle work and added home responsibilities and also spend time at the hospital supporting their loved ones.

Family and friends, naturally focusing on the needs of

"When my wife was going through treatment, I found it helpful to talk to a friend I trusted who was supportive and understanding of our situation. I was able to cry in this person's presence, and he helped me just by listening and letting me talk. I did not feel I had to be 'macho' through the whole ordeal, and I learned that it was most helpful to both my wife and me when I opened up about my feelings."

-Anonymous

"My significant other kept himself so busy during my treatment that he didn't have time to see me. It was his way of not dealing with the cancer.

"He didn't understand why our sex life had changed. I was always a very energetic person before the treatments, but during them, I had low energy. I had some difficulty convincing him it had nothing to do with him."

-Elizabeth, age 47

the woman with breast cancer, often forget this also is a distressing time for her husband or significant other.

Although support groups for spouses of women with breast cancer are almost unheard of, a kind word from a relative or friend can make a world of difference. Looking back, many husbands say they would like to simply have been asked, "How are *you* doing?"

Resuming Sexual Relations

Although most experts recommend sexual relations begin as soon as possible after surgery, communication is crucial. Many women fear rejection after surgery, particularly if they have had a mastectomy. Husbands, meanwhile, may be reluctant to approach their wives for fear they may cause them physical pain.

By refraining from physical intimacy, a husband may send a subtle message to his wife that her deepest fears about being unlovable and unattractive are true. The solution is simple: Retain a close bond by holding and caressing one another until the woman indicates to her husband that she is ready to be physically intimate. Generally, most women find their husbands to be loving, supportive and accepting of the situation.

Children - From Infants to Adults

The way a child feels about and understands the facts

surrounding his mother's breast cancer depends a great deal on his age. Yet it's essential that parents be truthful with children of all ages when discussing this disease, while at the same time telling them only as much as they want to know.

Even young children need to know why their mother is going to the hospital. Tell them as much as they can understand without overwhelming them. Most importantly, don't make them think you're keeping a terrible secret from them.

Children of all ages, even babies, pick up on their parents' emotions. They also are quite aware of phone calls and private conversations with friends. For this reason, it's important that family members share feelings.

Until the teen years, children think of their parents as all-powerful. Wanting to keep them in that role, they have trouble comprehending that Mom is sick and not as capable of doing things for them.

Following is age-specific information on helping children cope with a parent's breast cancer.

"My daughter and I had our best talks driving to and from school. I could casually direct the conversation toward her fears and questions, and it made us both feel better."

-Suzanne, age 50

Infants and Toddlers

Children this young benefit most from consistent schedules. Even infants and toddlers can benefit from their parents acknowledging their feelings. For example, tell a toddler: "Mommy will miss you. You might feel sad that I am gone for two days, but I will be back on Wednesday."

Provide the caregiver with a note regarding your child's

"One of the nicest things anyone did for me was when a neighbor contacted other neighbors and several friends and had a surprise luncheon for me at her house to celebrate my being done with treatment. As if this wasn't wonderful enough, they presented me with a generous gift certificate to a ritzy beauty salon for when my hair grew back."

-Marcia, age 44

schedule.

Young Children, Ages 3 to 6

Due to their less-developed thinking skills, young children do not understand the world the way adults do and therefore do not have the same worries. Concerned about the here and now, they are concrete in their thinking and have a limited perspective.

Children this age cannot reason and see things only from their points of view. Consequently, they may be more worried about missing a birthday party than their mother's surgery.

Because they often do not understand cause and effect, they think they somehow caused the cancer or that some strange event is responsible for it. They also may worry about catching or developing the cancer.

At this age, children fear separation more than death. Parents can dispel concerns by trying to maintain the child's daily routine. Experts recommend Mom make an audio tape of what will happen each day she is in the hospital. For example: "On Monday, I will fix breakfast for you and then you will go to school and Dad will take me to the hospital. That day, I will have the operation and feel sleepy. After school, Aunt Ellen will pick you up from school and give you a snack. Then Dad will pick you up and have dinner with you. Grandma will come stay with you while Dad visits me at the hospital. You and Grandma can read a book together and listen to our tape to see what you will do tomorrow. Grandma will put you to bed."

Other suggestions include writing the week's events on a calendar and making a booklet telling the story of "Mom Going to the Hospital and Coming Home." The child can draw pictures for the book.

Children who have not learned how to talk about their feelings and fears often express them by acting them out. Although they don't understand why they are upset and hurt, they may show these feelings by throwing temper tantrums, hitting and pushing others or withdrawing to their rooms.

Husbands and significant others should encourage children to express their feelings about Mom being in the hospital. Children should be reassured that they did not cause their mother to go to the hospital.

Elementary School Children - Ages 6 to 11

Although children this age are beginning to think more logically, they are still very concrete in their thinking and worry mostly about the immediate future. It is normal for them to feel their life is being disrupted by Mom's surgery. They also may feel they need to take responsibility for the family.

It is important to listen to their concerns and reassure

"I think being open with our kids was the best thing we could do. If you hide it from them, they just fill in the blanks with their imaginations, and that's probably worse. I didn't think my boys were too young at ages 8 and 10. I think they needed to face reality.

"My oldest son had to write a paper for school about what he would like to ask God for. He asked God that I not lose my hair when I was going through chemotherapy because he'd heard me say that was really important to me. He prayed every day that I not lose my hair, and I didn't."

-Dianna, age 33

"I've shared everything with my teenage daughter, and I have noticed something lately that I don't think she's even aware of. She's become very protective of me. She has to know where I am going and when I'll be home whenever I leave the house.

"I know she talks to her boyfriend a lot about it. But because I think she might have difficulty asking questions about my breast cancer, I just tell her."

-Faith, age 46

them that, for example, insurance will help cover the cost of surgery, and adults will be responsible for making decisions and caretaking. Let the child know it's OK to feel sad or angry about what is happening.

At this age, children are beginning to understand the finality of death and sometimes fear it.

Middle School Children and Teenagers

These children are going through rapid physical and emotional changes, so they are extremely vulnerable. Teenagers normally have a sense that they are immortal, and a parent's illness naturally alters this perception. Children in this age group are self-absorbed and have difficulty viewing parents as having needs.

Parents can help by sharing their feelings and listening to their teenager's feelings, if the teen is willing to share. Sometimes just hanging out together or chatting in the car is more effective than a serious talk.

Because teens are busy identifying their values, self-images, friends and goals, threatening to halt the process to help Mom during her treatment may be counter-productive. Teens may feel guilty while trying to simultaneously meet their parent's needs and their own.

Teenage Girls, Boys

Teenage girls also may feel at special risk for breast

cancer. Books such as "Relative Risk" address daughters of breast cancer patients and may be helpful. The "Every Woman's Risk" chapter at the end of this book also may provide some insight.

Teenage boys often become quiet and withdrawn when confronted with breast cancer, not knowing how to discuss what they consider a very personal part of their mother's anatomy. They may feel embarrassed talking about breast cancer because it deals with the breast, which they probably perceive as a sexual object.

Children of any gender and age can learn important coping skills by watching their parents support one another, and observing loving gestures from friends and relatives.

Grown Children

The term "child" is used because, when it comes to fears about losing their parents, grown children may become more childlike and needy.

Some grown children try to manage their mother's health care, while others deny she needs any support at all. Some telephone too much, others not enough. The best way to handle grown children is through open, honest communication. Tell them what kind of behavior is supportive and not supportive. The best way to get the support you need is to ask for it.

> "I finally had to tell my daughter I was not an old fogie and that I was quite competent to manage my affairs, but that I appreciated her concern."
>
> *-Priscilla, age 78*

Dealing with anger and other emotions

• Name the emotion

• Find a way of exploring the emotion

• Talk to someone

• Write down your thoughts and feelings

• Use music to express your feelings

• Shout it out

• Let it go (it takes up too much energy)

• Know that the emotion may come again, and it's OK to have emotions

• Be thankful for emotions

• Use your faith as a support

• Help others after you deal with your emotions

Friends and Other Family Members

Sometimes friends and family members such as siblings and parents are unsure how to handle a loved one's breast cancer diagnosis.

Parents usually are shocked to find their child is facing a possibly life-threatening situation. It is always difficult to consider losing a child. They may handle their shock in a variety of ways.

Some may overreact and try to control every facet of diagnosis and treatment. Others may deny the seriousness of the diagnosis and neglect to offer the support needed.

Siblings may feel threatened because their risk and the risk to their children is now increased.

Friends may be reluctant to contact you, fearing that a reminder of the breast cancer will upset you. Some women have been surprised to find close friends unable to deal with it at all, failing to call, write or visit.

Everyone copes with situations such as breast cancer in their own way. It's important not to take what seems like rejection personally.

On the positive side, many women have friends and relatives who come through with needed support, cooking meals, sending cards and listening patiently. New friends are often made through breast cancer support groups. Some women find these new friends give them more support and understanding than those they had been close to for years.

Your Rights At Work

Anyone who has had cancer is covered against discrimination in hiring, pay, promotion, firing, job training and job benefits by the Americans With Disabilities Act. The law applies to any private employer with 15 or more employees, as well as state and local government agencies, employment agencies, labor organizations, joint labor management committees, religious bodies that are also employers, and Congress. Federal government employees are covered by a different law.

For more information and an informative booklet, call the American Cancer Society at 1-800-ACS-2345.

"I have had the benefit of a death without dying. Instead of the person paying for my funeral receiving all the cards and flowers, I received them. I know how many people care; there were far more than I knew. This is a benefit I will carry with me for the rest of my life, no matter how short or long it might be."

-Sue, age 34

CHAPTER THREE

Surgery

Women diagnosed with breast cancer today have an advantage over their predecessors 25 years ago: They can choose from a variety of treatment options. Although a sign of progress, these options make the decision-making process painstakingly difficult for most women. Overwhelmed by unfamiliar medical terms and emotionally drained, they often go through the motions in a numb trance.

For this reason, experts advise women to take a friend or significant other along when interviewing surgeons, oncologists, radiation oncologists and other medical professionals. The friend also should take notes, as most women say later that little of what the doctors said registered at the time.

Differing Opinions

Medical oncologists, surgeons and radiation oncologists

"I consulted with four oncologists before making a decision about the removal of my breast. I went alone on each consultation, and this was hard. I was in school and so busy with classes that taking time to go to appointments put stress on me...

"It was hard to lose my breast, but better my breast than my life."
--Elizabeth, age 47

How To Know If You Have The Right Doctor

• Do you feel comfortable communicating with her?

• Is she gracious when you request a second opinion?

• Does she return phone calls as soon as possible?

• What is her experience in cases similar to yours? Is she board-certified in her specialty?

• How does she feel about pain control? Is she worried about dependency on narcotics?

• How does she feel about involving you and your family in the decision-making process?

• Does she take time to answer all of your questions?

don't always agree on the best course of treatment for their patients. Part of this stems from the unknowns which still surround breast cancer. For example, in one case two treatments may seem to have the same survival rate, while in another, two different doctors may strongly recommend opposite treatments.

Thankfully, as long as the tumor has been removed in a biopsy, most women can safely take a couple of weeks to interview medical professionals and research their particular type of cancer before making a decision. A reputable and qualified doctor will encourage patients to seek second opinions.

Mastectomy And Lumpectomy

Breast cancer surgery falls into two broad categories: **mastectomy** and **lumpectomy**. A modified mastectomy means the breast and some underarm lymph nodes are removed, while a lumpectomy means "breast conservation" - - the lump, some surrounding normal tissue and some underarm lymph nodes are removed.

Today, most women whose cancers are detected early can be treated without breast removal. In 1990, The National Institutes of Health (NIH) Consensus Conference provided sufficient evidence that, for the majority of women with early stage breast cancers, lumpectomy followed by radiation therapy has the same survival rate as modified

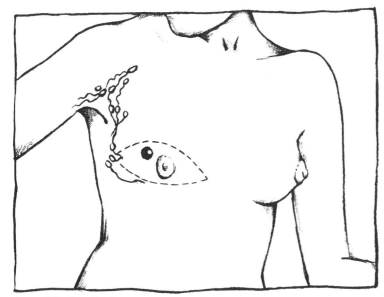

A modified radical mastectomy, which removes the breast, underarm lymph nodes and lining over the chest muscles.

mastectomy. Although controversy surrounding some studies which came to this conclusion raised doubts about the safety of lumpectomy, analysis without the controversial data revealed the same conclusion: Lumpectomy with radiation therapy is as effective as mastectomy for certain patients. Radiation after mastectomy may increase survival.

Still, mastectomy seems to be the No. 1 choice among women with breast cancer, particularly in the Midwest and South. Lumpectomies are more common in the Northeast and on the West Coast.

Following are the different types of mastectomy:

•**Modified Radical Mastectomy**: removal of the

Questions to ask your doctor before surgery

•Will I need a blood transfusion? Can I donate my own blood for transfusing?

•Will I need additional treatment with radiation therapy, chemotherapy or hormonal therapy following my surgery?

•Can breast reconstruction be safely done at the time of surgery or later? Would you recommend it?

•What side effects can I expect, and how long will I be hospitalized?

•Where will my surgical scars be?

•Will I have drainage tubes?

•How long will I be off work?

•Will there be any activity restrictions?

•When can I begin physical therapy?

"My doctors disagreed. My surgeon really wanted me to have a mastectomy, while my oncologist felt strongly about my not needing one. My gynecologist finally put it into perspective for me by saying that doctors are, for the most part, conservative on these issues, and if they are forced to make a recommendation, they'll usually say mastectomy. My oncologist said that if I were the type to lie awake at night worrying about it, I should have a mastectomy. But I knew I wasn't the type to worry like that, so I had a lumpectomy."

-Julie, age 38

breast; breast tissue extending toward the breastbone, collarbone and lowest ribs; **lymph nodes** in armpit; and sometimes the minor pectoral muscle.

•**Total or Simple Mastectomy**: removing only the breast.

•**Partial Mastectomy (or Quadrantectomy)**: removing only part of the breast.

Tumor size and location, tumor type, lifestyle, desire to preserve the breast and feelings about radiation therapy or chemotherapy all are factors to consider when deciding between lumpectomy and the different types of mastectomy.

Personal preference and lifestyle may steer women in one direction over another. For example, some women choose modified radical mastectomy with or without immediate reconstruction because they want to avoid six weeks of radiation treatment. Others choose lumpectomy because of their athletic lifestyles and/or desire to preserve their breasts. For women living in smaller communities, proximity to a radiation facility may pose a problem.

Analyzing The Facts

When determining which treatment option offers the best chance of survival, medical factors should precede everything else. Tumor management is, of course, the highest priority.

Several things may affect a doctor's recommendation for treatment. They include tumor size, whether there is lymph node involvement, whether the cancer has metastasized (spread), the type of cancer and the level of its aggressiveness. These factors also affect a woman's prognosis.

A lumpectomy typically can be performed on tumors up to two inches (five centimeters) in diameter. But if the tumor is large when compared with the size of the woman's breast, the best cosmetic solution may be mastectomy followed by reconstruction.

Any woman who is considering reconstruction should notify her general surgeon. Incision location is important, even if a woman has reconstruction years later.

Staging and Prognosis

Because breast cancers are detected at various growth stages, doctors use a staging process to determine each woman's prognosis and to guide further therapy.

The most widely used staging system, Tumor, Nodes, Metastasis (TNM), classifies breast cancers on the following basis:

T: Size and extent of the primary tumor.

N: Involvement of regional lymph nodes.

M: Presence or absence of distant metastasis.

The best prognostic indicator is the absence of lymph node involvement. While most surgeons still remove many lymph nodes in the armpit, a newer technique involves sampling a single node (the sentinel node) which avoids the

> "Our society is very hard on women's bodies. In American society, breasts sell everything. When you have a mastectomy, you really realize this."
>
> *-Faith, age 46*

> "Don't look in a mirror the first time. Look down instead, giving yourself time to get used to the effects of your surgery."
>
> *-Colleen, age 40*

side effects associated with the old procedure.

The sentinel node procedure involves identifying the first lymph node which drains the area of the tumor and examining it under the microscope. If that node is free of cancer, the other nodes do not need to be removed.

Because prognosis depends on so many different factors, a woman who has one or more less-favorable prognostic indicators should not be overly pessimistic. Many women who greet a poor prognosis with a positive attitude outlive their expected number of years. More importantly, breast cancer research is still relatively young, and current statistics are based on older studies. The more routine use of **adjuvant therapy** (chemotherapy or hormonal therapy) since 1988 promises more optimistic statistics for expected disease-free survival.

Following are the definitions for Stages 0 to IV. Describing patients' diseases in stages helps develop better therapies for the future by comparing outcomes.

Stage 0:   **Minimal Breast Cancer**
Carcinoma in situ: small tumor which has not invaded nearby tissues

Stage I: Small tumor, less than or equal to two centimeters (about one inch)
Negative axillary lymph nodes

No detectable metastases

Stage II: Tumor more than two centimeters but less than or equal to five (between one and two inches)

AND   Negative axillary lymph nodes

OR   Tumor less than or equal to five centimeters

AND   Positive axillary lymph nodes

BUT   No detectable distant metastases

Stage III: Large tumor (more than five centimeters) Tumor of any size with positive axillary lymph nodes fixed to one another or to other structures

BUT   No detectable distant metastases

A particularly aggressive form of breast cancer, **inflammatory cancer**, is classified as Stage IIIB. This usually is treated with chemotherapy before surgery.

Stage IV: **Distant metastatic disease**

Tumor of any size

Lymph nodes positive or negative

Cancer has spread to other body organs

OR   Tumor of any size with extension to

> "I had an uncle who was a doctor in New Mexico, and he told me years ago when he was dying, 'If breast cancer ever happens to you, have a mastectomy.' Now, I realize medicine has changed a lot in the past 11 years and this may be an outdated point of view, but what he said stuck with me, so I had a mastectomy for my own peace of mind."
>
> *- Marti, age 47*

> "I think I asked so many questions my doctors must have told me everything I needed to know. I wrote things down so I wouldn't forget them. Being well-rested made it much easier to face the challenges of each new day."
>
> *-Marcia, age 44*

chest wall or skin

OR   Tumor of any size with positive lymph nodes in the collarbone area

Hospital Stay

When packing for the hospital stay following surgery, include loose items which button down the front, because arm motion will be limited for awhile. Pretty nightgowns and scented toiletries make some women feel feminine and pampered after a mastectomy.

The length of a woman's hospital stay is determined by her treatment choice. For example, a woman who chooses lumpectomy with **axillary dissection** (the surgical removal of lymph nodes in the arm pit) can expect outpatient surgery and/or one night in the hospital. She most likely will need one drain inserted and one to two weeks recuperation time. Drains are thin tubes that extend from the surgical site to empty into a small bulb that is pinned to clothing. Drains prevent fluid buildup and infection after surgery. The amount of fluid gradually decreases over time as the wound heals. Drains are removed painlessly when drainage is minimal.

A woman who chooses lumpectomy with axillary dissection should have full range of motion in her arm within two to four weeks.

A woman who chooses a modified radical mastectomy without reconstruction, on the other hand, can expect one to two days in the hospital, one to two drains, two weeks recuperation and two to four weeks limited arm movement.

Some women find taping over the drain at the point of incision prevents tugging and lessens discomfort.

A modified radical mastectomy with immediate reconstruction will sometimes require more time in the hospital and a longer recuperation period. See the "Reconstruction" chapter for more information on this option.

Experts suggest a woman look at her incision before leaving the hospital. Some women like to have a significant other present. Most women do not find this as upsetting as they expected it to be. They are relieved to have their tumor removed, and this often outweighs the grief over losing a breast.

Straightforward Operation

Overall, breast surgery is a straightforward operation, with rarely any complications. Blood transfusions are usually unnecessary, although they may be required if a woman is having a mastectomy with immediate reconstruction. Many women prepare for this by donating their own blood in advance. As for pain, most women report little discomfort after breast surgery, other than that caused by drains and an incision in the armpit. Mastectomies can sometimes be

> "After my incision healed, I went out and bought a falsie. It was too uncomfortable - much too firm - so I did not use it. I found a pair of pantyhose, folded just right, worked quite well. As a joke, I gave the falsie to my husband."
>
> *-Carolyn, age 65*

"I love my mom no matter how many breasts she has. I'm just happy that she's OK."

- Gail, age 13

performed on an outpatient basis. Ask your doctor about this option.

Arm Mobility and Numbness

Following removal of the lymph nodes with either modified mastectomy or lumpectomy, the arm may be somewhat stiff for a few days to a few weeks. Easy stretching and pulling exercises should begin immediately to improve mobility, which ultimately will return to normal. Since no muscles are cut, strength also will return after recovery.

A skin nerve sometimes cut during lymph node removal may cause various sensations in the upper arm, including numbness and tingling, sharp pains or squeezing pressure, beginning a few days after the operation. These feelings usually subside within a few weeks. However, 2 to 3 percent of women may experience a chronic ache.

Phantom Breast

Up to 80 percent of women report feeling as if their breast were still present after mastectomy, similar to the perception of patients after amputation of a limb. If the tumor was painful, they also may be aware of sensations resembling that pain for weeks or months after surgery. Some women report sensations that come and go for years - not exactly painful, but reminiscent of their tumor. One woman reports feeling an ache in the area of her mastectomy whenever breast cancer is discussed. It may be comforting to know that bodily sensations can be recalled by the brain, and that not every pain in the area of surgery indicates a cancer recurrence.

Lymphedema

Some women later experience a persistent swelling in the arm caused by excess fluid that collects when the lymph nodes and vessels are removed. This condition is called lymphedema. It occurs in 5 to 10 percent of women after a mastectomy and usually occurs within three years. It also can occur after a lumpectomy with axillary node dissection.

While the causes of lymphedema are not certain, physicians often recommend the following in an attempt to prevent it:

- Lift nothing heavier than 10 pounds with the affected arm.
- Always wear heavy gloves and long sleeves when gardening to avoid cuts and thorns.
- Massage cream into cuticles daily to prevent hangnails.
- Never cut cuticles; gently push them back instead.
- Do not carry a heavy purse on the affected shoulder.
- Ask the doctor to describe post-mastectomy exercises.

For more information on lymphedema, call the National Lymphedema Network at 1-800-541-3259.

> "The doctor told us that after surgery I would not be able to lift anything over five pounds for six weeks. The night before I went in, I rocked my baby, who was 9 months old, for a long time and cried. I learned two things that night: I had to beat the cancer, and no matter what procedures I would have to face, nothing could be more difficult than that night."
>
> *-Kriss, age 38*

"After my diagnosis, I was amazed to learn that so many women I knew were breast cancer survivors. This, in turn, gave me a positive outlook on my future. If they beat this disease, I could, too!"

-Gina, age 50

Many women will notice a slight swelling of the affected arm after mastectomy. This is not necessarily lymphedema. If swelling, redness or warmth in the affected arm occurs, notify your doctor immediately. Infections in the arm can be serious and should be treated promptly.

Treatments for lymphedema include diuretics (water pills), compression devices (pumps that gradually move the lymph fluid from the arm), compression sleeves and massage therapy.

CHAPTER FOUR

Reconstruction

Just as early detection of breast cancer has dramatically improved in the past 40 years, so has breast reconstruction.

In 1990, members of the American Society of Plastic and Reconstructive Surgeons performed almost 43,000 reconstructions, an increase of 114 percent compared with the 20,000 procedures carried out in 1981. The reasons more women are seeking reconstruction include a change in perception and refined surgical techniques. Insurance companies typically will pay for breast reconstruction after mastectomy. Currently it is uncertain how health-care reform will affect this. The patient would be well-advised to check with her insurance company before any reconstruction is performed.

Today, most doctors agree that, as long as a woman is physically, psychologically and emotionally healthy, she can

"I would strongly recommend reconstruction to other women. It makes you feel whole again, and rebuilds your self-esteem."
-Diane, age 31

**Questions to ask
your doctor**

•**What are my reconstruction options?**

•**Which would you recom-
mend for me, and why?**

•**What are the side effects or
possible risks of each?**

•**Can you show me any
photographs of your work?**

•**When is the best time for
me to have reconstruction -
immediately following my
surgery or some time after?**

•**How does a reconstructed
breast differ from the real
thing?**

•**If I do not choose reconstruction, what are my other
options? What do you know
about prostheses or breast
forms?**

have reconstruction at any time — in many cases even during the same operative session immediately following the mastectomy.

Is Breast Reconstruction Right For Me?

It has been said that mastectomy treats the disease; reconstruction heals the mind. And most women who have undergone breast reconstruction would probably agree.

While women give different reasons for desiring breast reconstruction, most are concerned about body image. Many feel their breasts are an important part of their sexuality, while others desire reconstruction to erase the daily physical reminder of cancer. They also say breast reconstruction makes them feel whole again. Yet this in no way contradicts those women who feel quite whole without reconstruction. The decision is an extremely personal one.

Those women who do not opt for breast reconstruction may choose to wear an external prosthesis. Lighter and less bulky than in earlier years, today's prostheses can be worn as soon as a woman's mastectomy wounds have sufficiently healed. The "Breast Forms and Prostheses" section at the end of this chapter explores these options more thoroughly.

Some women are comfortable without a prosthesis or reconstruction. One woman diagnosed with breast cancer in her late 60s says reconstruction didn't seem important at the time of her surgery. She now wears a prosthesis, but just when she goes out.

Surgical Team Cooperation

Tumor management must be the foremost consideration for any woman diagnosed with breast cancer. The type and timing of reconstruction must be agreed upon by the medical oncologist, radiologist, breast surgeon and reconstructive surgeon.

For this reason, each woman's case should be reviewed by the breast cancer management team prior to treatment. If her physicians are certain she will need post-operative radiation therapy, reconstruction should be delayed until radiation is completed.

Whether a woman has immediate or delayed reconstruction, coordination between the surgeon and reconstructive surgeon is essential - not only to provide the best cosmetic result, but also to avoid creating a situation that might delay any **adjuvant therapy**.

Although both the surgical oncologist and reconstructive surgeon are primarily concerned with tumor management, the reconstructive surgeon will recommend placement of incisions which will optimize the final cosmetic result.

Immediate Vs. Delayed Reconstruction

Most women today are candidates for immediate reconstruction, which occurs immediately following a mastectomy

> **"The night before surgery, I was taking a walk with my 21-year-old son and telling him my fears and how I was going to be so scarred. He said, 'Those are battle scars, Mom, and you're going to win the battle.' I've never forgotten that."**
>
> *-Marti, age 47*

"It is great to live in a time where reconstructive surgery is an option and most insurance companies pay for it."

-Cathy, age 37

during the same operative session. The advantages of immediate reconstruction are:

●Economical: Both the mastectomy and reconstruction can be performed in the same surgery, lowering health-care costs.

●Emotional/Psychological: Many women are more emotionally comfortable waking from mastectomy surgery with a newly constructed breast.

●Personal: Women who are candidates for lumpectomy, but want to avoid the radiation therapy that accompanies it, may view mastectomy with immediate reconstruction as an alternative.

●Geographic: Women who live in rural areas, where radiation therapy is unavailable, may choose mastectomy with immediate reconstruction over lumpectomy and radiation treatment.

●Practical: Women who are career-oriented can alleviate time constraints and work-absence-related guilt by consolidating the two surgeries into one. Women with small children can avoid the inconvenience of having to schedule child-care arrangements around two surgeries.

As a general rule, immediate reconstruction allows for a better cosmetic result because the skin has not yet developed scar tissue.

But not every woman is a candidate for immediate reconstruction. Women with the following characteristics may need to delay reconstruction:

•Those who will need radiation therapy following mastectomy.

•Those who have advanced breast cancer.

•Those who are not healthy emotionally, psychologically or physically. Women under severe emotional strain due to other, unrelated problems are sometimes advised to delay reconstruction until their lives become more stable.

Immediate reconstruction is an option for women who are going to have chemotherapy.

Delayed Reconstruction

The biggest advantage of delayed reconstruction is time: For many women, the decision-making process for breast surgery alone can be exhausting. Delayed reconstruction gives them more time to consider their options and recover from the mastectomy.

Ideally, women who desire delayed reconstruction should tell their physicians prior to a mastectomy, because a strategically placed mastectomy incision can enhance the outcome of reconstruction.

Delayed reconstruction is recommended for women requiring post-operative radiation therapy or a bone marrow transplant.

"My husband was the one who really talked me into reconstruction. At the time, I just wanted to get it over quickly, but he thought I'd be so much happier with the way my clothes fit, especially being so active with swimming, volleyball and waterskiing. He thought being young I wouldn't want to mess with a prosthesis and some of the other things. I'm glad now that I had the implant."

-Dianna, age 33

"I was so in awe of the new breast my doctors had created for me that I showed it to almost everyone who came to visit me in the hospital. My elderly roommate found this rather disconcerting and told me so, but then added, 'Could I take a peek and see what all your girlfriends are oohing and ahhing about?'"

-Marcia, age 41

Reconstructive Options

Thanks to refinements in breast reconstruction techniques over the last 10 years, women can choose from a variety of reconstructive options.

Options include tissue expansion with **breast implants, back muscle (latissimus dorsi) flap, Transverse Rectus Abdominus Muscle (TRAM) flap** and **free flap**. All can be performed immediately following breast surgery or at a later date. Nipple and areola reconstruction are other, later, considerations.

Tissue Expansion Followed By Implant

More women opt for breast implants than other options, usually because they involve less surgery and recovery time.

Actually an internal prosthesis, the breast implant is inserted under the chest muscle, in a pocket created by the surgeon. But for most women, tissue expansion comes first.

Tissue expansion is a process whereby a temporary, expandable implant is placed underneath the remaining muscle and skin following a mastectomy. It can be placed during the same operative session as the mastectomy (immediate reconstruction) or after the mastectomy has healed (delayed reconstruction). This procedure generally takes one to two hours.

The tissue expander has a valve under the skin, which allows the plastic surgeon to add fluid each week, for about six to eight weeks, in order to gradually stretch the remaining skin and muscle. Some women report mild discomfort for 24 hours after fluid has been added.

Normally after six to 10 weeks, the expander reaches the desired size and can be replaced with a permanent implant. This procedure takes one to two hours.

If the patient needs a balancing operation on the opposite breast, a breast reduction or augmentation can be done at the same time. Performed properly, tissue expansion with placement of permanent implants can lead to a very acceptable breast reconstruction.

A few women, however, are candidates for an implant without tissue expansion. A woman with a relatively small opposite breast and enough tissue remaining on the reconstructive side would be a good candidate. This operation normally takes only one or two hours and, if done at the same time as a mastectomy, requires no additional hospital stay.

In the past, women have had two types of implants to choose from: silicone gel and saline.

Controversy over silicone-gel breast implants has led the Food and Drug Administration to limit their use. Currently, silicone-gel implants are available only for women who need or want them for breast reconstruction or for replacement of leaking silicone-gel implants already in place.

The only women who are not candidates for silicone-gel

"My 6-year-old daughter needed frequent reassurance that I would get better. She wanted to see the surgical results at all steps. While I was having reconstruction, she told people I was growing another breast. I had to tutor her several times about not talking about my body and respecting my need for privacy. It must have been hard for a 6-year-old."

-Ann, age 50

"During implant reconstruc-tion, I was uncomfortable sleeping on my stomach and one side. I learned to prop pillows at my back and under my arm to sleep more comfortably."

-*Suzanne, age 50*

breast implants are those seeking them for **augmentation** (breast enlargement) purposes only.

Saline implants, which are widely available, are filled with salt water, much like the body's own fluids. Any type of implant can develop a capsular contracture (hard scar). In this situation, the body develops a layer of firm tissue around the implant. The breast may become firm to the touch. Leakage of saline implants can happen 2 to 5 percent of the time. This can lead to deflation and replacement with a simple outpatient procedure.

Women frequently choose saline implants for breast reconstruction. They are an attractive option for those concerned about the controversy surrounding silicone-gel implants.

Women who choose breast implants generally have rounder, firmer breasts, as opposed to breasts that match their natural shape. Although implants don't feel as natural as breasts reconstructed from a woman's own tissue, they require much less surgery and recovery time than the other options.

Infection is another possible complication from the implant procedure. In such cases, the expander or implant is removed until the infection has healed, and then is rein-serted.

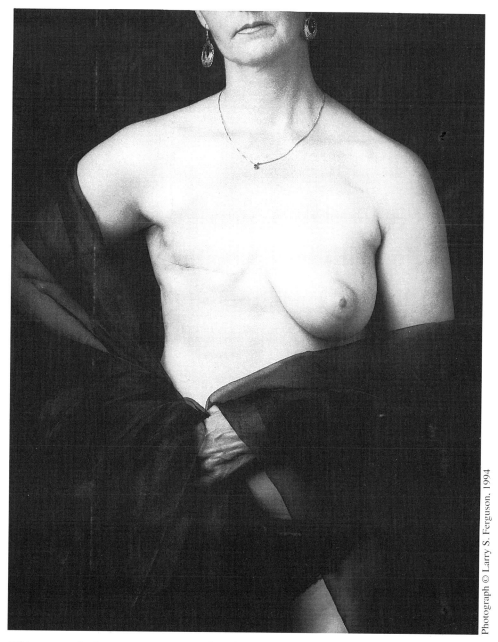

This woman had a mastectomy at age 43. She is planning to have reconstruction.

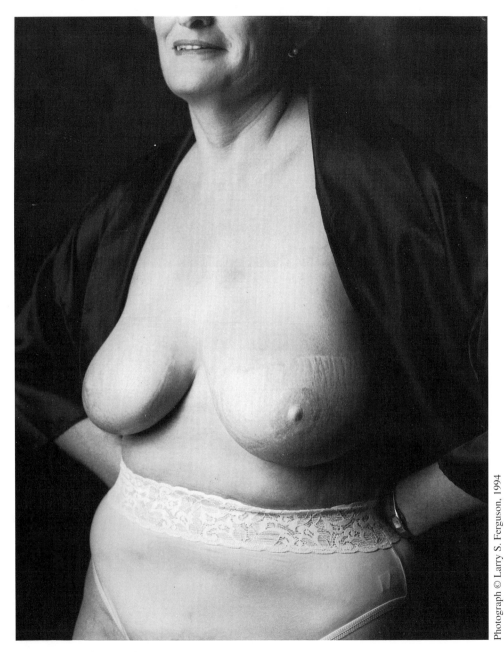

Both of this 47-year-old woman's breasts were removed. She chose bilateral (two-sided) TRAM Flap (or tummy tuck) reconstruction, followed by nipple and areola reconstruction.

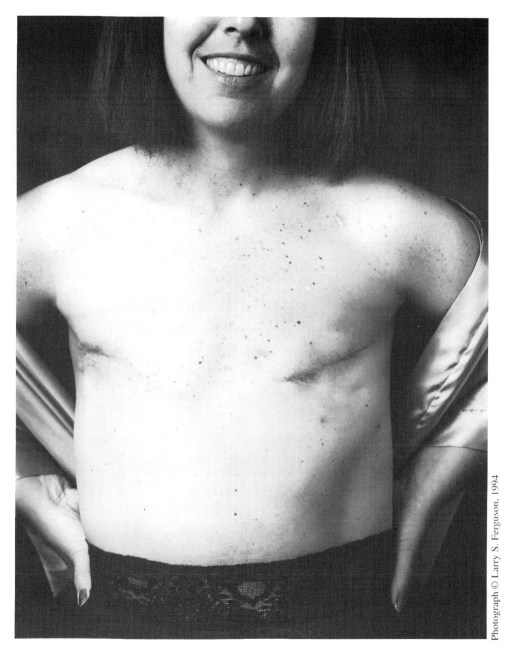

Bilateral mastectomy. This 37-year-old woman has decided against reconstruction.

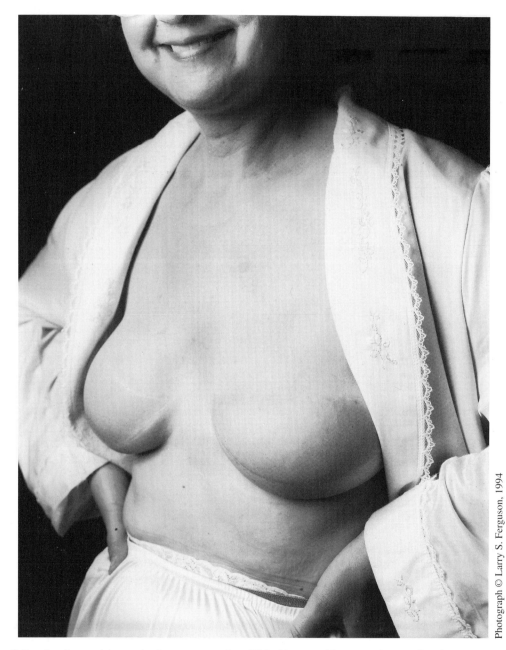

Saline implants without nipple reconstruction. This 50-year-old woman is not planning nipple and areola reconstruction, which requires a second operation.

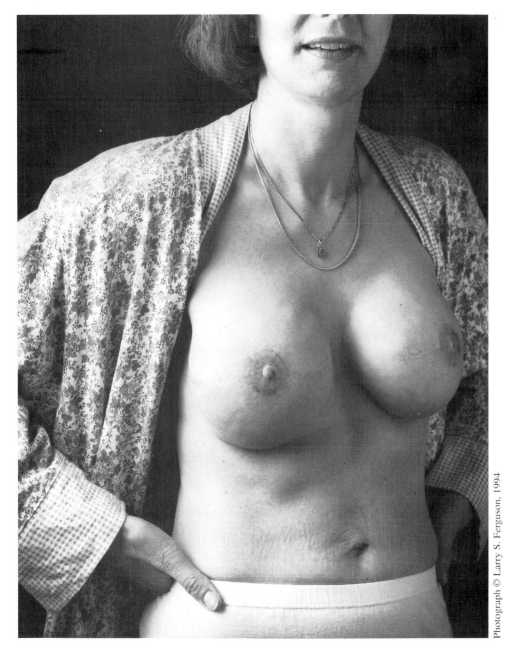

Tissue expanders with saline implants, followed by nipple and areola reconstruction. This woman was 38 at the time of her surgery.

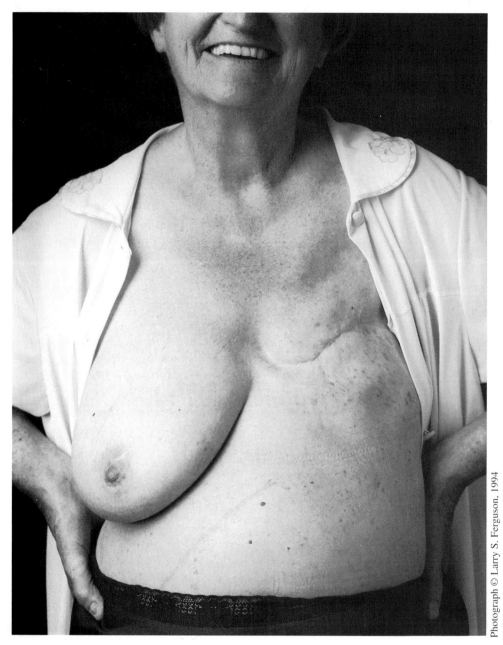

Simple mastectomy without reconstruction. This 70-year-old woman says she never considered reconstruction. She sometimes wears a prosthesis.

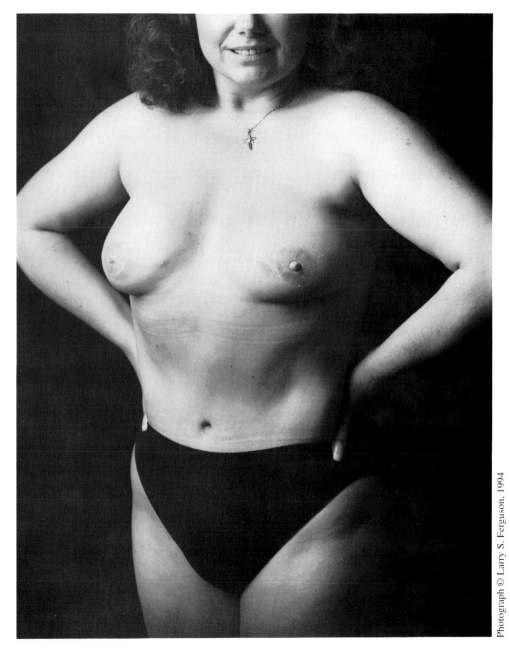

Bilateral mastectomy followed by immediate TRAM Flap reconstruction. The nipple and areola were added later. This woman was 38 when diagnosed with breast cancer.

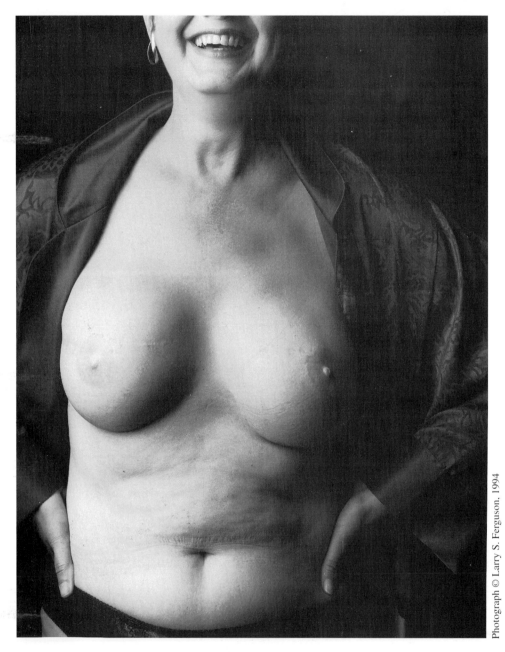

Tissue expanders were inserted immediately following this 46-year-old woman's mastectomy. Saline implants were placed six weeks later, and nipple and areola reconstruction followed.

"Tummy Tuck" and Other Options

Increasing in popularity are procedures that allow women to have their breasts reconstructed from their own tissue. Although tissue also is available from the buttocks, outer thighs and back, by far the most common source for obtaining tissue is the lower abdomen.

The TRAM flap operation is nicknamed the "tummy tuck breast reconstruction" because the skin and fat transferred for breast reconstruction is the same tissue removed during a so-called tummy tuck.

Breast reconstruction with the tummy tuck procedure usually takes between four to six hours of surgical time. Recovery time also is longer than that needed for a breast implant. Normally, full recovery takes six to eight weeks.

The procedure involves transferring the abdominal tissue up to the chest wall, while maintaining a healthy blood supply to keep the tissue alive.

The skin and fat of the lower abdomen remain attached to the lower end of a narrow muscle that runs from the rib cage to the pelvic bone. A tunnel is created between the absent breast area and lower abdomen, and the skin and fat tissue is then delivered up to the mastectomy site. The delivered skin and fat is then tailored and sculpted to most closely resemble the opposite breast. Because abdominal fat is similar in consistency to that of a normal breast, a new breast can be reconstructed which looks and feels very natural. A

> "For me, immediate reconstruction with the TRAM flap was an easy choice to make, because I was the perfect candidate for it. I found my consultation with the plastic surgeon pretty fascinating and wonderful, especially seeing photographs of the ones after a year. The ones right after surgery were kind of upsetting."
>
> -Marti, age 47

"Unlike some of the women I've gotten to know, I can wear all my pre-mastectomy clothes. I can throw on my clothes and not have to wonder if everything is 'on straight.' And no special bras. I'm not saying reconstruction is the answer for everyone, but it was for me. I'd do it again in a minute."

-Marcia, age 44

breast constructed from this tissue will respond to changes in weight along with the rest of the body.

Because women sometimes require a blood transfusion during this operation, it is recommended that they donate their own blood in advance.

Advantages to this procedure are a reconstructed breast that looks and feels more like a natural breast, and something similar to the cosmetic "tummy tuck," or flattening of the lower abdomen. Although major complications are infrequent, they include infection, loss of skin and fat if the blood supply is interrupted, and bulging of the lower abdomen if a hernia develops.

Women with the following characteristics may not be candidates for TRAM flap reconstruction. Those who:

- are very thin or obese;
- have abdominal scars from a previous surgery;
- are heavy smokers;
- suffer from diabetes or other blood vessel disease; or
- have pre-existing lung or heart disease.

Other "Flap" Options

Other "natural tissue" reconstructive options include using the back muscle flap and flaps from the buttocks and thighs. Both typically are used only when tissue transfer from the abdomen is not possible.

The back-muscle flap is otherwise referred to as the

latissimus dorsi myocutaneous flap - a triangular-shaped back muscle. During reconstruction, this muscle carries the skin needed to replace tissue removed during the mastectomy.

The muscle and overlying skin is detached from its connecting points and then transferred to the front of the chest through a tunnel created underneath the skin. Once it is brought to the front, the skin is sutured into place and a breast implant is used to create the volume of the breast.

A new technique uses fat from the back to match the breast that was removed. In this case, skin with enough fat and underlying muscle can be used to mold a breast shape without a breast implant. Application of this particular technique is quite limited, however.

Nipple and Areola Reconstruction

Whether a woman opts for implants or tissue reconstruction, she typically must wait six to eight weeks for nipple and areola reconstruction. Because cancer cells can be found near the nipple, saving and using the nipple and areola from the removed breast is not an option.

Several nipple reconstruction methods exist. Most commonly, the nipple is created from skin and fat of the central portion of the reconstructed breast.

The areola can be reconstructed with a skin graft from the abdomen or inner thigh. Both the nipple and areola can

"When I had my nipple reconstruction, the plastic surgeon put EKG electrodes on my chest to indicate nipple placement. My reaction was, 'This looks great, I'll just go home now.'"

-Nancy, age 51

"I don't know if it has something to do with age or what, but it (reconstruction) just didn't seem that important. The surgeon said there would be an imbalance, but I don't find that at all.

"I didn't even know what a prosthesis was. I had the idea it would be something like a brace, with steel and all. But it's quite soft, and you just pin it to your brassiere. It doesn't move at all, it's very comfortable. I was well-endowed, and I'm pleased with it."

-Monica, age 70

be tattooed for a good color match, if necessary.

These procedures can be performed on an outpatient basis, using local anesthesia.

Breast Forms or Prostheses

There are many attractive alternatives for the woman who does not desire reconstruction after mastectomy. A volunteer from "Reach to Recovery" can visit either before or after surgery to present the options. Located through your surgeon or hospital, many of these volunteers are long-term breast cancer survivors. Most women with newly diagnosed breast cancer find this experience reassuring and encouraging. Volunteers can demonstrate breast form or prosthesis options, and can discuss the pros and cons, costs and where to purchase them.

Recent years have witnessed the introduction of breast forms which are not only more convenient and comfortable, but also closer in size, weight and appearance to the remaining breast than older breast forms. Examples include Discrene and Amoena. Both attach to the chest wall with the help of a small piece of Velcro-like fabric that can remain painlessly in place for several days or weeks. Another product, the "Softee," is a post-surgery undergarment, with a prosthesis, designed to be worn home from the hospital.

Benefits of Reconstruction

Many women say breast reconstruction:

•Restored the most visible symbol of their femininity.

•Helped to dissipate the daily reminder of breast cancer.

•Gave them another option: Rather than lumpectomy followed by radiation treatment - a good, breast-conserving option - they could choose mastectomy followed by breast reconstruction.

• Lessened the fear of disfigurement once associated with cancer therapy.

Breast reconstruction improves the lives of many women who are diagnosed with breast cancer. Although all breast reconstruction options require the investment of additional recovery time and expense, most women say the benefits far outweigh the inconveniences.

"Reconstructive surgery is an individual choice. However, I feel strongly that recovery is a mindset in which this restorative surgery played a role. The daily reminder of a scar where a once cancerous breast had been was gone. In its place not only appeared a new breast, but also aspects of my personality that had vanished with a diagnosis of cancer. To my reconstructive surgeon at every visit I give a roll of Lifesavers, appropriately renamed 'Soulsavers.'"

-Sue, age 34

CHAPTER FIVE

Radiation Therapy

In use since the 1920s, radiation therapy has been used to treat women who have had lumpectomies, or have had mastectomies, but a large number of nodes were involved or the cancer had invaded the chest muscles.

New research indicates radiation after mastectomy — regardless of node involvement — improves survival.

Radiation therapy is recommended for most lumpectomy patients because, without it, the risk of recurrence is unacceptably high. Radiation therapy can reduce that risk three to four times. Combined, lumpectomy and radiation therapy can obtain results comparable to mastectomy.

Like chemotherapy, radiation kills cancer cells. The difference is that chemotherapy treats the entire body, while radiation therapy treats only the affected area.

"For some reason, radiation therapy terrified me the most. Now I don't know why, because going through it actually wasn't so bad."

-Terri, age 38

Questions to ask your doctor

• How will radiation therapy improve my chances for survival?

• How long will each treatment take?

• How many times will I need radiation?

• Who will administer my radiation treatments?

• Where will my treatments be administered?

• Should I bring a friend, or can I come alone?

• What are the possible side effects of radiation therapy? What are the long-term side effects?

What To Expect

Most women start radiation therapy about two weeks after surgery. Your surgeon should forward copies of your pre-operative mammogram, test results and pathology report to your radiation oncologist.

The purpose of the first visit is to pinpoint the area receiving radiation. The area will be marked in water-soluble ink or tiny tattoos. The ink may wash off when bathing. If the marks begin to fade, notify your physician so they can be reapplied. Ink will eventually fade, but tattoos are permanent.

Some women report that radiation therapy is a dehumanizing experience. The combination of being marked with tattoos and having to remain partially nude during treatment can cause emotional discomfort. Warning of these procedures in advance seems to help.

Radiation therapy treats the whole breast - the area which would be removed in a mastectomy. Usually, localized radiation also is administered to the area where the tumor was located. The lymph-node-bearing regions are occasionally treated, as well.

Treatments, lasting a matter of minutes, are given every weekday. The entire process can last from five to six weeks.

Side Effects

Because it is administered only to the affected area,

radiation therapy's main side effects usually are limited to that area, with a few exceptions.

Possible side effects include:

•swelling of the area;

•redness resembling a sunburn;

•fatigue;

•blotching of the skin or dilated blood vessels in the treated area, which may persist; and

•soreness with swallowing.

Radiation therapy is not thought to adversely affect a woman's fertility, menstrual periods or reproductive system. Some women have even breast-fed their babies with their other, untreated breast.

While some cosmetic side effects can occur, most are minor and vary from woman to woman. They may include a slight discoloration of the skin and a somewhat firmer than normal breast. Occasionally, the treated breast may become slightly smaller or larger.

Experts advise taking special care of oneself during radiation treatment. They recommend women:

•Get plenty of rest.

•Treat skin gently, using lukewarm water and mild soap to wash the treated area.

•Wear loose, comfortable clothing.

•Don't use any powders, creams, lotions or deodorants on the area without first consulting the radiation oncologist.

"All my doctors were willing to talk to all my family and friends. No matter who I brought with me, they talked to them.

"When I felt sick from the radiation, I had a different friend go with me every day, and he talked to every one of them."

--Linda, age 47

> "I was going to school during my treatment, so I would nap on campus on a small couch in one of the bathrooms. I would curl up with my alarm clock set and sleep. I had various reactions from people in and out of that bathroom."
>
> -*Elizabeth, age 47*

•Avoid exposing the treated area to the sun. Some physicians recommend wearing protective clothing or using sunscreen for up to one year following radiation treatment.

•Don't try to scrub or rub off the marks or tattoos. The ink marks eventually will fade on their own. Tattoos, however, are permanent.

The Right Physician

It's important that women considering radiation therapy see a board-certified **radiation oncologist**. It's also important that the treatment be administered by a certified **radiation technologist**, under the supervision of the radiation oncologist.

Some women who live in rural areas and desire a lumpectomy choose to spend the weeks of radiation therapy with a friend or relative who lives near a quality facility. The facility should have treatment-planning computers, as well as trained physics and dosimetry personnel to calculate dosage. This treatment usually is delivered utilizing a linear accelerator.

To locate the nearest licensed facility, call the Cancer Information Service (CIS) of the National Cancer Institute (NCI) at 1-800-4-CANCER.

CHAPTER SIX

Adjuvant Therapy

While surgery treats the tumor, **adjuvant therapy** — **chemotherapy**, **hormonal therapy**, or both — treats the whole body. Aimed at killing undetectable cancer cells left in the body, these anti-cancer drugs disrupt a cancer cell's ability to grow and multiply.

Many women who have a mastectomy also will have adjuvant therapy, particularly if there was lymph node involvement. Although exceptions occur, pre-menopausal women typically are given chemotherapy, while post-menopausal women are given hormonal therapy. A combination of both may work best for some women.

When tailoring a treatment plan for a particular patient, an oncologist will consider her risk, the size of her tumor, the aggressiveness of the tumor, any lymph node involvement, her risk of recurrence and other parameters discussed in

"My son, age 9, and I were discussing how chemo-therapy works and how I would be bald in the near future. 'Will you get a wig?' he asked. I said, 'Yes.' He responded with, 'OK, but don't get a red one, it's not your color.'"

-Marcia, age 41

Questions to ask your doctor:

• How soon should treatment begin?

• How long will my treatment last?

• Who will be responsible for administering my treatment?

• Where will my treatments be administered?

• Should I come alone, or bring a friend or relative along?

• What are the risks and possible side effects of my treatment?

• What symptoms should prompt a call to you?

• Can I continue my normal activities, such as working and exercising, during treament?

chapter one. For example, a small cancer that is non-invasive has such a low risk of **metastasizing** (spreading to other body organs) it may not require adjuvant therapy. On the other hand, an invasive tumor larger than one centimeter may require adjuvant therapy, even if there is no lymph node involvement.

Because the risk of cancer spreading is gauged in part by the presence of cancerous cells in the armpit lymph nodes, women with node involvement are almost always advised to have adjuvant therapy. However, since 1988, when the National Cancer Institute issued a clinical alert statement that all premenopausal women, regardless of nodes, should consider adjuvant treatment, doctors have been recommending it to women without node involvement, as well. Recent studies have shown that adjuvant therapy can extend survival in these women, too.

Although adjuvant therapy usually follows surgery, it is sometimes administered beforehand to shrink a tumor before surgery. It is then called **neoadjuvant therapy**.

You And Your Doctor

It is important that you feel comfortable with your **oncologist**. She should be available when you need to talk, and should be willing to answer all questions.

Remember that doctors are people, too. Like you, they have unique personalities and communication styles. If you are uncomfortable with your doctor's particular style, choose another doctor.

To ensure the best possible treatment, come to each appointment prepared with questions. It also helps to bring a written list of all your medications, including birth control pills, vitamins and herbs. Even over-the-counter drugs, such as aspirin and ibuprofen, are important for your doctor to know about.

Although patients sometimes become frustrated when they have to sit in the waiting room, it's important to remember that emergencies do occur. If waiting irritates you, call ahead of your appointment and ask if your doctor is on schedule.

You also can arrange to get your blood tests done a few days ahead of time so the results will be ready to discuss with your doctor the day of your appointment.

The Drugs

Most chemotherapy drugs are given intravenously and by mouth, while **hormone drugs** typically are taken by mouth. Both treatments should begin within four weeks of surgery, or as soon as a woman's incisions have healed.

Many women are concerned about how **chemotherapy** drugs - which destroy cancer cells - affect healthy cells. Although some normal cells are damaged in the process, cancer cells are much more sensitive to the effects of chemo-

"I didn't want to go through chemo; I didn't want to lose my hair. But if there's a chance that there's some of it (cancer) left in my body and chemo would take care of it, that six-month inconvenience was worth it. And that's what I tell everybody.

"I've heard gals in my support group say they're not going to bother having radiation or chemotherapy. That's your life you're playing with, and if that's going to bring that percentage down, then you've got to do every-thing you can to make sure you did. It's a life or death situation, it really is."

-*Dianna, age 33*

> "Family members and friends lent me scarves and hats to wear when my hair fell out. I was constantly reinforced about my appearance because of these hats and scarves."
>
> *-Elizabeth, age 47*

therapy than are healthy cells. In fact, because chemotherapy damages all fast-growing cells, certain body cells also will be harmed, such as the rapidly growing cells of the hair and gastro-intestinal tract.

Somewhat less concern surrounds the drugs used in hormonal therapy, because they work to prevent tumor growth rather than damage cells in the rest of the body.

Intravenous Catheters

Drugs given by vein may be administered either through a vein in the arm or via a surgically implanted catheter, or tube. This tube is inserted into one of the large veins near the base of the neck and remains attached in place until chemo-therapy is completed. A surgeon can place it in an outpatient procedure.

Two major types of devices allow access to veins: external and internal. This access allows delivery of chemotherapy in a convenient and reliable fashion and allows easy and pain-less access for blood samples. External catheters are called either Groshong or Hickman. Internal catheters are called ports. Ports lie under the skin while external catheters exit the body in the mid-chest region. Ports allow for activities such as swimming.

Insertion of Groshong, Hickman and ports are outpa-tient procedures which require minimum care. They are removed in the doctor's office.

Discuss the risks and benefits of this method of administering chemotherapy with your doctor.

Dosages

Chemotherapy dosages are determined individually, and doctors strive to give the highest dose possible without harming the patient. Chemotherapy drugs can be taken daily, weekly or monthly.

Hormonal therapy typically is taken by mouth. Tamoxifen (Nolvadex), the most commonly used hormone, usually is taken in two daily doses of 10 milligrams each. The dose can vary, depending on the hormone.

Tamoxifen (Nolvadex)

Tamoxifen is an anti-estrogen drug which blocks action of the estrogen in cells. However, it acts very much like estrogen itself in heart and bone tissue. So while it may cause some menopausal symptoms, such as vaginal dryness, fatigue, depression, hot flashes, weight gain and insomnia, it also can protect against osteoporosis and coronary artery disease. Memory loss also is seen with tamoxifen use. However, this may not be directly related to the drug but to menopause, which is known to be accompanied by memory loss. A similar drug, Raloxifene, is also being studied.

An increase in uterine cancer has been seen in a small number of women who take tamoxifen for more than five

> "I worked during all six months of my chemotherapy. I just shortened my hours by one quarter. I got more tired as my counts dropped further and further down with each cycle of chemotherapy. But I'd do it again in a minute."
>
> -Suzanne, age 50

> "Losing my hair was very painful. All I could think about was how long it takes a baby to get a full head of hair. I thought it would be years before I would have as much hair as I had lost. Wrong: It grew back much faster than I had expected. Six months after my last treatment, I got a perm. What a great day it was when I saw hair on my head."
>
> *-Fran, age 47*

years. Liver cancer has been reported in rats which were given high doses of tamoxifen, but risk of the disease for women has not been proven. Tamoxifen also may have an effect on eyes, so regular examinations with an ophthalmologist are recommended. Ask your doctor about your risk for these illnesses, as well as a thorough list of possible side effects. A generic form, called tamoxifen citrate, is available.

Other Drugs

The usual first-line chemotherapy drugs used in adjuvant treatment of breast cancer usually are given in combinations of cytoxan, methotrexate and 5-FU (CMF) or cytoxan, adriamycin and 5-FU (CAF). Prednisone and tamoxifen also may be given with these regimens.

Following is more specific information about each drug.

•cyclophosphamide (Cytoxan). Often given daily by mouth for two weeks out of every four, Cytoxan is best taken in the morning with lots of water. Drink at least 8 to 10 glasses of water daily while taking this drug to flush it rapidly out of the bladder and prevent irritation. If allowed to concentrate, Cytoxan can cause bladder cancer, but this is rare. Other possible side effects include nausea, vomiting, loss of appetite, menstrual irregularities, low blood counts and hair loss. A slight chance of liver problems and infertility also exist. This drug also can cause temporary lactose intolerance, which means mik and dairy products are poorly digested, resulting in gas, diarrhea or intestinal discomfort.

•methotrexate. Given intravenously, methotrexate can cause sores in the lining of the mouth, throat and bowel. If you notice any bleeding in stools or undue soreness swallowing, notify your doctor. Other side effects may include nausea, vomiting, sun sensitivity, low blood counts, eye inflammation and stomach ulcers. In rare cases, this drug may cause hair loss, headaches, liver problems, blurred vision and lung problems.

•5-fluorouracil (5-FU). This drug is given intravenously and can cause extreme sensitivity to the sun. Use a good sunscreen, such as Shade UVA Guard SPF 45, before your chemotherapy session and throughout treatment months. If you are sensitive to the chemicals in sunscreens, try Neutrogena Chemical-Free Sunscreen.

Other side effects may include mouth sores, nausea, vomiting, diarrhea, low blood counts, loss of appetite, hair loss and sore throat. Rarer side effects include rashes, nail changes and darkening of the skin.

•doxorubicin (Adriamycin). Given intravenously, Adriamycin usually is given to women whose tumors were negative for estrogen receptors. Some studies have shown this drug to have higher activity against breast tumors. It may be substituted for methotrexate in cases where a more aggressive treatment plan is indicated.

Side effects include hair loss, mouth sores, nausea,

"Chemo was relatively easy on me. I was careful to follow instructions, and my family was considerate of my lack of energy. I purchased a good wig the same color as my hair, and for the most part, we continued our social life when we felt like it. A good sense of humor really helps!"

-Carolyn, age 65

Insurance frequently covers high-dose chemotherapy with bone marrow rescue (transplant). This is offered to women with 10 or more positive lymph nodes as standard adjuvant therapy. Even women with four to nine nodes are now eligible for the same protocol.

> "My oncologist laughed when I told him I quit my job because I had to have breast surgery and chemo. I said, 'What?' And he said, 'Well, gee, life goes on.'"
>
> *-Dianna, age 33*

The new dose-intensification protocol currently under study uses six cycles of chemotherapy for 18 weeks for women at high risk for recurrence. No increased vomiting is seen with this protocol.

vomiting and low blood counts. It also can cause nail and skin darkening and liver problems, but these are rare. Another side effect of this drug is toxicity to the heart muscle, but the doses used in breast cancer treatment are calculated to cause the least damage and the greatest good. This list of side effects is not exhaustive. Ask your doctor for other possible reactions, and always report anything unusual.

Other treatment agents are used for different types and stages of breast cancer. They include Navelbine, Gemzar, Arimidex, Taxotere and Herceptin.

Side Effects of Chemotherapy

Hormonal therapy has few troublesome immediate side effects. The side effects of chemotherapy, however, are widely known. Most patients are anxious about chemotherapy's side effects, and worry about losing their hair and getting sick.

It helps to remember that the side effects are only temporary. They also vary widely from person to person. Just because an acquaintance had problems with nausea and hair loss doesn't mean you will. Many side effects can be controlled by well-regulated drug dosages and schedules. And there is usually no pain associated with chemotherapy.

Most importantly, the unwanted side effects of treatment must be measured against the medicine's ability to destroy the cancer.

The most common side effects of chemotherapy are low blood counts, nausea, hair loss and fatigue. Some women also experience the symptoms of menopause.

Blood Count

Red cells, which carry oxygen and thus give the body fuel for energy, can become low during chemotherapy, leaving you fatigued and a bit short of breath on exertion. White cells, which are important in fighting infection, also can become low. Doctors watch carefully for this with blood tests every two weeks or so. Your doctor will hold off treatment or lower your dosage if your white count gets dangerously low, and may even recommend an injection of a growth factor (Neupogen) that causes bone marrow to produce and release more white cells to fight infection. This should enable you to keep to your normal chemotherapy schedule.

Any signs of infection should be reported promptly to your oncologist. Symptoms may include fever, redness, pain or swelling. Platelets, the cells that help blood clot, also can become low, causing you to bruise easily. If this happens, or if unusual bleeding occurs, notify your doctor.

Nausea

While not completely eliminated, most nausea can now be controlled either by over-the-counter preparations or drugs prescribed by a doctor. Various medications can

> **"I used to whip off my wig on the hot drives home from work and enjoy the astonishment on the faces of the other drivers."**
>
> *-Suzanne, age 50*

"When I found out chemo-therapy would cause me to lose my hair, the news was almost as devastating as finding out I had cancer. My daughter and I went to the wig salon and were surprised to find so many styles, colors and shapes to choose from. I found one that matched my color and style, and one month later my friends and co-workers were marveling at how real it looked. The only thing missing was a few gray hairs."

-Dianna, age 47

be injected or given by mouth to prevent nausea and vomiting in most patients. Those who do experience nausea say it usually lasts a day or two and then subsides.

Eating small amounts of food at a time, eating slowly and eating dry foods such as toast or crackers may help. Avoid eating a heavy meal immediately before treatment.

Hair Loss

Because chemotherapy treatments vary, side effects also vary from person to person, so not every woman undergoing chemotherapy loses her hair. Hair loss can begin within a few days or weeks of treatment, but usually starts about three to four weeks after treatment begins. Some women experience no more than thinning and greater hair loss when brushing, combing or washing their hair.

But just in case, experts advise buying or reserving an attractive hair piece that not only matches your hair color but also your hair style - *before* you begin treatment. Being prepared makes the adjustment somewhat easier. Wigs should be cut and styled to match your look.

Women who feel uncomfortable wearing wigs have turned to other options, such as turbans. A supply of decorative scarves breaks up the monotony and adds color. Like the other side effects, hair loss is only temporary.

Regrowth usually is complete within three to five months after chemotherapy. Some women note beginning regrowth of brows, lashes and hair before chemotherapy is complete. The "Look Good... Feel Better" program matches women with cosmetologists who provide free advice on makeup and wigs. For more information, call 1-800-395-LOOK or your local American Cancer Society office.

Fatigue

Many women - including those who feel some fatigue - continue working during chemotherapy treatment. Those who experience fatigue say the first day after treatment is typically the most difficult, and it gets better from there. A flexible schedule and understanding employer helps, though, as some women find themselves tired late in the day. A nap at home before dinner is recommended.

Fatigue may increase as the months of chemotherapy progress, and may persist for a year or two after treatment ends.

Menopause

Some women stop menstruating during chemotherapy, and also may experience sweating and "hot flashes" similar to those experienced during menopause. Other symptoms related to menopause include vaginal dryness, night sweats, fatigue, depression, insomnia and weight gain.

While younger women usually will begin menstruating again after chemotherapy, women closer to 40 may not. For

"My hair loss was harder on my husband than it was on me. The morning most of it came out, he was still asleep. When he awoke after I had left for work and saw all the hair in the waste-basket, he cried."

-Gina, age 50

> "Although I felt sick during much of my chemotherapy, I felt it was an insurance policy. If my cancer were to return, I had done everything available."
>
> *-Sue, age 34*

those who resume menstruating, fertility is not thought to be adversely affected.

Some women misinterpret symptoms they experience as a result of chemo or hormonal therapy as a sign that their cancer is returning. It is important to discuss all symptoms and fears with your doctor. Educating yourself through reading about adjuvant therapy, cancer and menopause may answer questions and bring greater peace of mind. See the resources list at the end of this book for suggestions.

Prevention Is Key

Adjuvant therapy is recommended for women with breast cancer because it can prevent a life-threatening recurrence. It's important to remember that women don't die from cancer in the breast, but from cancer that has spread outside the breast. By reducing the risk of recurrence for thousands of women, chemotherapy and hormonal therapy help save lives.

CHAPTER SEVEN

Risk of Recurrence

For the woman diagnosed with breast cancer, the risk and worries don't end after treatment. Most women worry about cancer recurring or developing in their other breast, and about the risk for their daughters, sisters, granddaughters and other female relatives. See chapter eight for information on hereditary risk factors and the risk for all women.

Fear of Recurrence

Universal to every woman who has received a diagnosis of breast cancer is the fear of its recurrence. For many, this fear first surfaces when the initial shock of diagnosis has worn off, and surgery is complete. Some, on the other hand, don't begin to confront their fears until chemotherapy or

> "I've been told there will come a day when I don't think about breast cancer the minute I open my eyes in the morning. I look forward to the day I won't worry about breast cancer recurring any more."
> *-Shari, age 52*

Questions to ask your doctor:

•What type of breast cancer did I have?

•Based on my diagnosis, what is my risk of recurrence?

•If I do have a recurrence, how will you treat it?

•How does my risk of recurrence differ from my risk of getting a new breast cancer?

•What is the risk for my daughters, sisters, mother and other female relatives?

•Based on my family history, do I have familial or hereditary breast cancer, and, if so, how should my family members protect themselves?

•What is my risk of developing a new cancer?

radiation therapy is complete, when frequent visits to familiar doctors and nurses end. Feeling strangely vulnerable, they may begin to fear recurrence on a daily basis. Every small headache or bodily pain may be experienced with a wave of anxiety, accompanied by a certainty that the cancer is back.

Thankfully, women report that these feelings subside with time. Soon, they can go entire days without thinking of breast cancer or worrying about its recurrence, breathing easier with each checkup until two years, then five, have passed.

Although breast cancer has been known to recur as late as 25 years after diagnosis, most recurrences occur within the first five years, and especially the first two. After the 10-year mark, a woman's chance of recurrence is very small.

Risk of Recurrence

The same tumor characteristics that are used to guide therapy also are used to predict the risk of recurrence. They include tumor size, lymph node status, tumor receptors for estrogen and progesterone, DNA ploidy and S-phase studies. Ask your doctor about your specific risk, but keep in mind these are only relative indicators and should not be thought of as absolutes. Most tumors posses a mixture of both "good" and "bad" characteristics, making predictions of a cancer's behavior difficult. Living each day with hope and a positive attitude can go a long way toward redeeming a less-than-positive prognosis.

Follow-Up Care

Your doctor will see you every month or so until all your blood counts stabilize after chemotherapy. He may ask for blood tests with every visit until he is satisfied that all is normal. He may also begin to monitor for possible recurrence, using the bloods tests CEA, CA 15-3 or CA 27-29. These tests are used by some physicians to follow their patients. If a persistent elevation is noted in one or both tests, it may indicate recurrence. Because they are useful in following a known recurrence and its response to therapy, the use of these tests before recurrence is controversial.

Your doctor also may have you undergo periodic screening tests, such as a chest X-ray, bone scan and liver scan. These tests are best used only if symptoms exist, so many doctors normally do not order them otherwise. Diagnosing a recurrence with these tests before any symptoms are noted has not been shown to prolong survival.

As more time elapses after completion of treatment, your doctor will lengthen the intervals between visits. For example, you may see your doctor every month for a while, then every three months for two years, every four months for the next three years and, finally, every six months. This schedule varies according to each woman's individual needs.

Of course, self-examinations and mammograms remain

> **"Even today when I hear about a friend or acquaintance recurring with the disease, my emotions turn to fear, sadness and anger."**
> *-Lorraine, age 48*

"There is a common thread that is often woven throughout the lives of the many who have done far more than survive cancer. There is truly a devotion to the enthusiasm of living."

-*Sue, age 34*

critical. Women treated by lumpectomy should focus on both breasts, while those who have had a mastectomy should care for the remaining breast, also examining the incision, collarbone, armpit and chest wall for thickness or lumps. If found promptly, a local or even regional recurrence of breast cancer may not shorten your life. Local recurrence after lumpectomy is treated and staged as if it is a new, primary cancer. The risk of recurrence is greater in the first five years.

Thankfully, drugs also are showing promise in preventing recurrence. Tamoxifen, which is used to treat patients with estrogen-positive tumors in one breast, also prevents tumors from occurring in the other breast for many of the women who take it. The study begun in 1992 was halted due to the positive role of tamoxifen in breast cancer prevention. Tamoxifen's side effects can include hot flashes, depression, blood clots, cancer of the uterus, eye problems, memory loss and weight gain. Development and use of drugs like Tamoxifen but with fewer side effects is ongoing.

Women who want to take an active role in preventing a recurrence sometimes turn to simpler strategies, such as eating nutritious foods, gradually resuming a daily exercise program and setting aside time each day for quiet meditation. Some studies actually link a survival benefit to a low-fat diet, exercise and meditation. If nothing else, these activities improve quality of life.

Risk of a New Breast Cancer, Other Cancers

Many women feel, at least unconsciously, that if they have had breast cancer they no longer have to worry about cancer. Unfortunately, they may then neglect examining the opposite breast after mastectomy, or the same breast after lumpectomy.

The risk of developing an entirely new breast cancer in the opposite breast is about 0.5 to 1 percent per year after diagnosis of the first breast cancer. Some women with high-risk cancers may have increased risk both in the operated breast after lumpectomy and in the opposite remaining breast.

Hereditary Cancer Syndromes

Having breast cancer may increase a woman's risk of developing other cancers if her breast cancer was part of a hereditary syndrome. Related cancers include colon cancer, cancer of the pancreas, lung cancer, ovarian cancer, lymphoma and prostate cancer in men.

A new hospital-based computer program can analyze a woman's family history to determine if she is at risk for other cancers. This computer program, distributed by OncorMed, can be installed by any local hospital. For more information, call the Hereditary Cancer Institute at 1-402-280-2942.

Chapter eight includes more detailed information about the risks for hereditary cancers.

"I used to be in a high hover for two weeks before my checkups, worried about what my tests would show. Now, two years later, I only worry for a day or so."

-Phyllis, age 40

> "It was much harder for me the second time around. We discovered a tumor in my other breast one year after I finished chemo for my first breast cancer. So I did it all again - surgery and chemo. One year later, I've put it all behind me."
>
> *-Jill, age 48*

If Breast Cancer Recurs

No one wants to think about the possibility of cancer recurring, but for most women, it is impossible not to. When fear of recurrence immobilizes you, call your doctor and check it out. Physicians are accustomed to handling these fears and would rather you talk to them than worry silently at home.

If breast cancer recurs, it may do so in the large bones of the body. This can cause pain which at first may seem to come and go. Areas such as the hips, thighs, shoulders, spine and ribs are affected.

Breast cancer also can recur in the lungs, which usually shows up on a chest x-ray or as a dry cough, and rarely as shortness of breath. It can recur in the brain, manifesting as a persistent headache. Brain recurrence also can show up as numbness or tingling, or as a loss of vision. When breast cancer recurs in the liver, symptoms usually do not manifest themselves until the liver is extensively involved. Blood tests may detect liver recurrence before symptoms, such as jaundice or pain in the right upper abdomen, reveal themselves.

Fear of recurrence leads most women to become quite anxious before each follow-up visit to their oncologists. Over time, these feelings subside.

If breast cancer recurs, treatments exist to put it into remission. Chemotherapy, hormonal therapy and bone marrow transplant are available, as well as the hope of new, innovative therapies. Radiation therapy is used to ease the pain of bone metastases, or spread of tumor to the bone.

Many women live years after diagnosis of breast cancer recurrence. Although cure of breast cancer after recurrence is rare, new chemotherapies, immune therapy and new gene therapies may halt the spread of metastases and change the future of breast cancer recurrence. In any event, recurrence does not mean sudden death.

"We all grieve if one of us recurs. But strangely, these women and their courage are the ones that give us the most strength and hope."

-Kate, age 55

CHAPTER EIGHT

Every Woman's Risk

Over the years, experts have identified specific factors which may put women at increased risk for breast cancer. Yet, because most breast cancer patients are female, the No. 1 risk lies in simply being a woman.

Because every woman is at risk for breast cancer, the absence of other specific risk factors should not preclude precaution: All women should practice monthly breast self-examinations and have a baseline mammogram between ages 35 and 39, followed by mammograms every year after age 40.

Average Risk For All Women

Breast cancer is perhaps the most-feared disease among women today. Although heart disease kills 10 times as many

"My daughter wrote a beautiful tribute to me a year later, when she had to write a paper on a signficant event in her life. Until then, I hadn't realized what an impact my breast cancer had on her."

-Donna, age 45

> "It took a minimum of three months to where I was pretty comfortable with my life again. And I remember telling my doctor at the time, 'I think I'll go back to my volunteer work.' He said that was the best thing I could do. I find it's so much better to keep busy than think so much about my health."
>
> *-Monica, age 70*

women as breast cancer kills, most women consider breast cancer a more frightening disease. The statistics bear witness to the thousands of lives breast cancer touches each year.

In 1970, American Cancer Society statistics reported one woman in 16 would develop breast cancer throughout her lifetime. By 1993, after several revisions, the numbers were one in eight. Without a clear understanding of the significance of these numbers, the average person may conclude that breast cancer is reaching near-epidemic proportions.

While not discounting the severity of this life-threatening cancer, it is important to remember that these statistics refer to **lifetime cumulative risk.** This means that if all the individual yearly risks were added together, a woman who lived to age 85 ultimately would have a one in eight chance of developing breast cancer.

When the numbers are broken down, the average woman has about a 1 percent risk of developing breast cancer between ages 35 and 45. Between 35 and 55, she has a 2.6 percent chance. As she approaches age 85, the individual yearly risks add up to about 12 percent. As a woman grows older without a breast cancer diagnosis, her lifetime cumulative risk actually decreases. However, women between ages 50 and 70 have a greater risk of developing breast cancer than they had between 35 and 45.

Most studies suggest risk factors for breast cancer are not even additive, let alone multiplicative. In other words, a woman who has two risk factors - such as a premenopausal mother with the disease and never having had children - does not necessarily have a risk that is the sum of the two or can be multiplied by two. More importantly, all known risk factors combined account for only 30 percent of all breast cancer cases. In other words, 70 percent of all new breast cancer patients have no identifiable risk factors.

Still, the following known risk factors are significant. Every woman should be aware of them.

Gender and Age

Two predominant factors which seem to predispose people to breast cancer are gender and age. The disease primarily affects women, although about 1,400 American men were diagnosed with breast cancer in 1996.

The longer a woman lives, the greater chance she has of getting breast cancer. Women over age 50, for example, have a much higher incidence of breast cancer than younger women. Twenty-seven women out of 100,000 will be diagnosed with breast cancer at age 30, according to the National Cancer Institute. About 212 women out of 100,000 will be diagnosed at age 50, and 404 out of 100,000 will be diagnosed at age 70.

"My mom has breast cancer, but I never really worry about getting it myself."
-Natasha, age 19

"I'm terrified of getting it, but I don't want to worry my mother with this."
-Jill, age 17

Seventy percent of all new breast cancer patients have no identifiable risk factors.

Flaws in genes are also called "mutations."

Many women fear insurance discrimination as a result of genetic testing for the breast cancer gene. National legislation to prevent discrimination against those who test positive for genetic disorders will be enacted in July, 1997.

Family History

Among the most widely recognized risk factors for breast cancer is family history. Of the 180,000 cases diagnosed in the United States each year, as many as 10 percent stem from hereditary defects. Experts now believe that 90 percent of inherited breast cancer can be traced to flaws in two genes, which they call Breast Cancer 1 (BRCA1) and Breast Cancer 2 (BRCA2). Flaws in BRCA1 involve families with breast cancer only, breast and ovarian cancer and colon and prostate cancer. BRCA2 flaws involve breast cancers, very few ovarian cancers and most male breast cancers. The flawed gene can be inherited both from female and male relatives.

A flaw in BRCA1 is associated with early-onset breast cancer and ovarian cancer. Flawed BRCA2 is linked to early-onset breast cancer and a higher incidence of breast cancer in males, but not to ovarian cancer. A person who carries one of the genes would have an 85 to 90 percent risk of developing breast cancer. Tests to determine which members of cancer-prone families carry either gene are now available.

A hospital-based service which addresses these issues is presently distributed by OncorMed to help local hospitals across the country evaluate a person's potential to develop any kind of hereditary cancer.

OncorMed's computerized genetic risk-assessment system collects, with a woman's consent, the cancer history of her family, including first-degree relatives, which are parents, siblings and children, and second-degree relatives, which are grandparents, aunts, uncles, nephews and nieces. A team of hereditary cancer experts then evaluates family members' risks for hereditary cancer. The system also provides physicians with expert advice on diagnostic and preventive care for women with the potential of developing breast or other cancers. For the nearest hospital with access to OncorMed services, call the Hereditary Cancer Institute at 1-402-280-2942.

The following chart illustrates the risk of developing breast cancer among all women compared with the risk of developing breast cancer for women with the flawed BRCA1 gene at various ages:

Age	% among carriers	% among all women
40	16	.5
50	59	2.0
60	77	4.0
70	82	7.0
80	86	10.0

It is hoped that further research will reveal a simple blood test for women whose relatives have breast cancer to gauge their own risk.

Statistically, the odds of getting breast cancer are two to three times as high for a woman whose mother or sister had the disease, and the risk is even higher if that relative devel-

"My mother died of breast cancer at age 32, when I was 7. As I approach 30, I am becoming more aware of my own risk for breast cancer.

"My sister and I talk about it a lot. We know we should do breast self-exams, but we're unsure of how to do it and what to look for."

-Cindy, age 28

"When I asked an aquaintance who had also had a mastectomy how she was doing with her therapy, she said, 'My God and I can handle anything that is thrown our way. I'm just waiting for what's up next so we can get on with the game plan.'"

--Roxanne, age 52

oped breast cancer before menopause or had cancer in both breasts. Possibly up to 10 percent of all women with breast cancer have **true hereditary breast cancer**. In these cases, there is a definite genetic transmission in a dominant mode for the development of breast cancer. Typically, these women develop breast cancer at an early age and have bilateral disease.

Those shown to have the gene defect face up to an 80 percent breast cancer risk by age 65. These are families which have members in many generations with breast and other cancers, such as ovarian.

About 20 percent of women with breast cancer have what is termed **familial breast cancer**. Familial breast cancer is a tendency toward the development of breast cancer in families without a definite genetic predisposition. This may be due to the fact that women in particular families have a greater percentage of body fat or have their first pregnancies later in life. It may be this sharing of characteristics that put each generation into a higher risk category.

One study of 117,000 women over 12 years showed invasive cancers developing in 2,389 women. Women who had neither a mother or sister with breast cancer had about a 7 percent chance of getting it from ages 30 to 70. The likelihood rose to about 10 percent for women whose mothers had breast cancer after age 60 and to 12.5 percent if the mothers were stricken before age 50.

The risk for a woman whose sister had breast cancer was about 13 percent, and rose to 17 percent if both a sister and mother had it.

However, findings from the Harvard University Nurses Health Study indicate that having a close family member with breast cancer is not as ominous as once thought. This study found that women who have a mother or sister with breast cancer have a risk of developing the disease by age 70 that is only 2.5 times greater than the average woman.

Some doctors advocate mastectomy for any woman who sees two immediate family members develop breast cancer before menopause. In a 1992 survey, physicians at the Johns Hopkins School of Hygiene and Public Health found that 90 out of 700 Maryland surgeons had performed at least one preventive mastectomy.

Onset of Puberty

Women who started menstruating before age 12 are 20 percent more likely to develop breast cancer than women who were 14 or older at first menstruation. Early puberty is believed to correlate with higher levels of circulating estrogen over a woman's lifetime. Estrogen increases the risk of breast cancer because it supports the growth of many breast tumors.

Delayed Childbearing and Breast-feeding

When compared with women who have their first child

"My mother's breast cancer helped me to become more aware of breast cancer. The risks and also the great possibility of survival became apparent to me."

-Gail, age 13

> **"When I was first diagnosed, I questioned whether I was strong enough to fight the battle. Now, I'm amazed not that I made it, but that I ever doubted my strength."**
>
> *-Kriss, age 38*

before age 18, a woman who is 30 before giving birth has four times the risk of breast cancer. Women who have never borne children also are at increased risk. Estrogen is a factor here, too.

Women who begin breast-feeding at age 19 and continue nursing at least 18 months reduce their premenopausal risk of breast cancer by 50 percent.

Onset of Menopause

Women who reached menopause after age 55 have double the breast cancer risk of those whose last period occurred before age 50. Considering a woman's entire menstrual and reproductive history, the common denominator seems to be the number of ovulatory periods a woman experiences during her lifetime. Those who get their first periods at an early age and experience menopause late in life, with no interruption of the estrogen-progesterone cycle with pregnancy, seem to harbor the greatest risk.

Fat Intake

Although definitive proof of a link between diet and breast cancer in humans is still lacking, several studies show populations with greater fat intake have a higher incidence of breast cancer.

In Japan in 1959, for example, the average person's diet contained 23 grams of fat per day. In 1973, this had risen to

52 grams. During this period of time, there was a 30 percent rise in the incidence of breast cancer. Japanese women who move to the United States also have an increased breast cancer risk.

It has been suggested this may not result entirely from increased fat intake. Japanese women typically eat a diet higher in cruciferous vegetables, including cabbage, broccoli, cauliflower and bok choy, which contain a compound that deactivates estrogen by breaking it down to a form unable to fuel tumors. It is possible that these women not only increase their fat intake when moving to the United States, but also decrease their intake of these cruciferous vegetables.

In animal studies, scientists have shown that dietary fiber also can reduce the risk of breast cancer, perhaps by influencing the body's metabolism of estrogen. Studies on human populations support the idea: Even though fat intake is similarly high in the United States and Finland, breast cancer rates are lower in Finland, where fiber consumption is high.

Other studies suggest vitamins A and C and beta-carotene may protect against cancer. And more than 100 studies have shown significant decreases in cancer rates among people whose diets are high in the fruits and vegetables that contain these vitamins.

Body Shape and Size

Body shape and size seems to have some influence on the

> **"One of the positive things that came out of my diagnosis was that it helped my stepdaughter realized how much she cared for me. It enhanced our relationship."**
>
> *-Gina, age 50*

"Still think about it? It never leaves my mind. But I have learned a few things. Don't accept anything at face value, and never stop asking questions. It's just too critical to let someone else make these kinds of decisions for you."

-Faith, age 46

risk for breast cancer. Postmenopausal obesity, for example, increases the risk of breast cancer and its recurrence. In a study of women with breast cancer headed by Dr. Ruby Senie of the Centers for Disease Control, 32 percent of obese women (at least 25 percent above optimal weight) developed cancer recurrences, compared with 19 percent of normal-weight women.

It also is thought that the distribution of fat has something to do with the incidence of breast cancer. Women who have higher concentrations of fat in their upper- and mid-torsos have a higher incidence of breast cancer than those with "pear shapes." Pear-shaped women have a greater concentration of fat in the hip and buttock regions.

Abdominal fat cells, which are larger and more metabolically active, are thought to convert certain compounds into circulating estrogens. This is usually not the case in the fat found in the hip and buttock region.

Cigarette Smoking

Although for years smoking has been noticeably absent among the risk factors for breast cancer, a recent study suggests smoking may escalate a woman's risk of dying from the disease.

Smokers were 25 percent more likely than non-smokers and ex-smokers to die of breast cancer, according to a 1994 American Cancer Society survey of 604,412 women who were initially free of cancer. The risk grew with the number of cigarettes a woman smoked, culminating in a 75 percent greater risk among women who smoked two packs a day or more. Quitting seemed to return a former smoker's risk to that of a lifelong non-smoker.

Researchers say the study does not suggest smoking causes breast cancer. They believe the increased risk may stem from poorer survival or delayed diagnosis.

Alcohol Intake

Some studies suggest the risk of breast cancer is increased if alcohol (beer, wine or liquor) is consumed more than twice a week.

Radiation

Exposure to x-rays is known to cause breast cancer. The developing breast tissue of young women is thought to be especially susceptible to x-rays. For example, radiation therapy for an enlarged thymus gland (a gland in the neck area), which used to be performed on infants, is now known to cause an increase in breast cancer risk years later.

In the past, tuberculosis was treated with x-rays, as was mastitis, an inflammation of the breast sometimes associated with nursing. Scoliosis used to be followed with x-rays, and an increase in breast cancer incidence occurred.

Even today, young women who have survived a child-

> **"My 10-year-old son heard me say once, 'Why did God do this to me?' And he said, 'Mom, God must not have wanted you yet. Otherwise, he wouldn't have let you find the lump.'"**
>
> *-Dianna, age 33*

"Once I was eventually told about my stepmother's cancer, I never thought for one moment that she wouldn't be able to beat it. The fact that she was really honest about how she felt day-to-day and after treatments really helped. I respected that honesty.'"

--Tim, age 16

hood cancer can trace the development of breast cancer back to a treatment which included radiation to the chest area. Mammography only involves exposure to about 1/4 rad, which is about the same amount of radiation one is exposed to on a cross-country airplane trip. Older mammography units used doses as high as four or nine rads. Between 10 and 500 rads are considered a high enough dose to cause cancer to develop. The lag time between radiation exposure and development of cancer is about 10 or 20-plus years.

Birth Control Pills

A great deal of controversy surrounds the risk of birth control pills in relationship to breast cancer. A recent study demonstrated no increased risk.

Hormone Replacement Therapy

Hormone replacement therapy after menopause or removal of the ovaries is common. Yet, as with birth control pills, whether or not these hormones increase breast cancer risk is still unclear. Studies are now underway to determine if replacement hormone therapy is safe for breast cancer survivors.

Environmental Agents

Pesticides and herbicides, especially those which are chlorine-based, promote breast cancer by acting as estrogen.

DDT, lindane and heptachlor have been banned in Israel, and a marked drop in breast cancer mortality has been noted. Atrazine and arachlor, still used in this country, also have been implicated in promoting breast cancer. Some researchers are even investigating certain plastics in which food is stored or cooked, since some plastics are known to mimic estrogen.

Benign Breast Disease

Specific forms of **benign breast disease** can predispose women to breast cancer. Most women with "lumpy" breasts do not have the atypical changes that predispose them to cancer. Diagnosis of this condition requires a biopsy and a pathologist's examination of the tissue.

If the pathologist sees **atypical intraductal hyperplasia** (a growth of abnormal cells within the milk duct), the woman will have an increased risk of developing breast cancer. It is commonly thought that atypical intraductal hyperplasia increases a woman's risk of breast cancer by about 1.96 percent.

Hope For The Future

Because it takes 10 to 20 years to develop meaningful statistics on the benefits of breast cancer treatments, mortality hasn't changed much in 50 years. In the last 10 years, however, since the start of adjuvant therapy for node-nega-

"After the mastectomy, I was advised to have my other breast removed and reconstruction started. One of my daughters asked me after my second mastectomy what they found, and I replied that they hadn't found anything wrong. My 8-year-old piped up, 'Are they going to sew it back on?'"

-Gayl, age 45

"I don't think people can really understand statistics, concerning cancer or anything else, until they are a statistic.'"

--Melissa, age 18

A flawed BRCA1 gives a woman an 85 percent risk of developing breast cancer, and a 40 to 66 percent risk of developing ovarian cancer. Males with the flawed BRCA2 gene have a 6 percent risk of developing breast cancer.

tive breast cancer and bone marrow transplant for advanced disease, we are beginning to see an increase in survival. It is thought that in years to come chemotherapy will be considered a crude tool in cancer treatment. Instead, treatment of breast cancer likely will include use of various immunotherapies. In fact, researchers are now developing breast cancer "vaccines" to prevent metastasis, as well as other therapies which use the body's own immune system to combat the disease.

Earlier detection also will be a reality, not only through techniques such as digital mammography and Miraluma, which can see tumors in the dense breasts of younger women, but also through blood tests, which will reveal cancers too small to detect by any other method.

For the small group of women who are genetically predisposed to breast cancer, genetic testing is currently available.

In light of these medical advances, there is much room for optimism. For many women, there is a realistic hope for survival and cure of breast cancer. Even women who experience a recurrence can survive and enjoy quality living.

We hope that in the future, breast cancer will be considered no more than a chronic disease women live with and keep under control, like high blood pressure. Women eventually may recall the days of surgery and chemotherapy for breast cancer as primitive. We are truly on the brink of a new age in cancer detection and treatment.

Studies are currently underway which place viral particles into tumor cells and then give the patient aggressive anti-viral treatment, which kills the virus and the tumor. Drugs that boost the immune system's functioning also are being used. Anti-blood vessel growth treatments which stop tumors from spreading are being developed, as well.

For those of you who have read this book because you already have been diagnosed with breast cancer, please know that our thoughts and prayers are with you, as you begin living the rest of your life after breast cancer. Survival is probable. Not just five-year, disease-free survival, but bounce-the-grandkids-on-your-knee survival. In fact, your life can and should be more than just survival. Triumph over your fear and you can live a wonderful, love-filled life despite - and maybe because of - a diagnosis of breast cancer.

"There is no caliber of words to describe the euphoria of regaining one's life. And for most, there is life after breast cancer. After the long uphill climb through treatment and surgeries, the tremendous view from the top is very much enjoyed."

-Sue, age 34

In Good Company
(an inner dialogue)

"What do you mean, it was cancer?
(I am too busy for that)

"Yes, I'll be there in the morning"
(I don't mind losing a breast)

"Please turn the morphine pump higher"
(Oh my God, this really hurts)

"Your chemo will last only six months"
(Oh, well, a baby takes nine)

"Is that a wig? You look stunning!"
(Surely he's flattering me)

"Welcome: Breast Cancer Support Group"
(I am in good company)

- Suzanne W. Braddock, 1993

Thanks

Dr. Margaret Block and Dr. Bob Langdon, Jr., for their expertise on chemotherapy; Dr. Patrick J. McKenna and Dr. Janalyn Prows for their contributions to the Radiation Therapy chapter; Dr. Henry Lynch and Dr. Ramon Fusaro for the section on hereditary breast cancer; Dr. John J. Heieck and Dr. Richard J. Bruneteau for their invaluable assistance in the reconstruction of patients photographed in chapter four; Mollie Foster, Ph.D., for her contributions to the Coping chapter; Judy Dierkhising, Ph.D., for her input on dealing with the emotional needs of the breast cancer patient; members of the Nebraska Methodist Hospital Breast Cancer Support Group for their comments, wit and strength; and Sue Kocsis, a real spark, whose encouragement meant so much.

The authors also are deeply grateful to the women who answered personal and sometimes painful questions in order to help others. Their comments, present on nearly every page of the book, taught us how strength and hope can triumph over despair. Although we could not use every comment, each was deeply appreciated.

To the women who shared their surgery and reconstruction in photographs, a very special thank you. What a wonderful gift to give every woman considering these procedures. We are indebted to photographer Larry Ferguson for his creativity and sensitivity in portraying these women not as medical results but as real, living women.

Thanks, too, to the many other physicians, patients and friends who contributed in direct and indirect ways to this book. All were motivated by the uniform desire to help women conquer breast cancer.

Glossary

A

adjuvant therapy: chemotherapy, hormonal therapy, or both.

anesthesia: a procedure in which a patient receives medications that block out pain. General anesthesia causes loss of consciousness.

anesthesiologist: a medical doctor specially trained to administer anesthesia.

aneuploid tumor cells: cells which have abnormal amounts of DNA, a less-favorable prognosis and are more aggressive.

aspiration: a procedure in which a hollow needle withdraws fluid from a breast mass into a syringe or vacuum tube.

atypical intraductal hyperplasia: a growth of abnormal cells within the milk duct.

augmentation: the method of enlarging one breast so it matches the other.

axilla: armpit

axillary dissection: the surgical removal of lymph nodes in the armpit.

B

benign breast disease: noncancerous breast conditions.

biopsy: removes tissue from the suspicious area so it can be examined under a microscope.

bone marrow transplant: removal and later reinfusion of bone marrow to allow for toxic chemotherapy

bone marrow: soft cell tissue in the bone center, where red and white blood cells are manufactured.

breast cancer 1 (BRCA1): a gene used to track hereditary breast cancers.

breast implant: a saline- or silicone-filled device that is placed underneath the skin and made to look like a breast.

breast reconstruction: the method of reconstructing a breast after a mastectomy.

breast reduction: surgery to diminish breast size.

C

cancer: a general term for diseases characterized by uncontrolled, abnormal growth of cells that can invade and destroy healthy tissue. Also called malignancy.

chemotherapy: anti-cancer drugs which disrupt a cancer cell's ability to grow and kill cancer cells left in the body.

clustered microcalcifications: a group of small, white dots which show up on a mammogram.

D

DNA: what genes are made of.

delayed reconstruction: when breast reconstruction after mastectomy is delayed for weeks, months or even years.

diagnosis: process of determining the nature of a lump.

diploid tumors: made up of tumor cells which resemble normal breast cells in DNA content.

ductal breast cancer: starts in the milk ducts.

E

early detection: the cancer is small when it is detected - usually no larger than two centimeters in diameter - and has not spread to the lymph nodes around the breast.

estrogen: a female sex hormone produced by the ovaries, adrenal glands, placenta and fatty tissues.

excisional biopsy: a type of open biopsy in which the tumor is small and completely removed.

expander: an empty sack placed behind the chest muscle and filled with saline over a period of months to stretch the skin before a breast implant is put in place.

F

free flap reconstruction: a method which uses a woman's buttock and/or thigh tissue to reconstruct her breast after mastectomy.

frozen section: part of the biopsy tissue that is immediately frozen. A thin slice is later mounted on a microscope slide and examined by a pathologist.

H

hormonal therapy: the use of hormones to prevent tumor-cell growth.

I

imagery: a method of relaxation which involves visualizing the body healing cancer cells. Also called visualization.

immediate reconstruction: when breast reconstruction is performed immediately following mastectomy, in the same surgery.

incisional biopsy: a type of open biopsy performed if the tumor is large, and only a small piece is removed for examination.

inflammatory breast cancer: a particularly aggressive form of breast cancer usually treated with chemotherapy before surgery.

in situ: the cancer has not spread through the wall of the milk duct, where it originated.

invasive: the cancer has spread through the wall of the milk duct, where it originated, into the surrounding breast tissue.

L

lattisimus dorsi flap: a breast reconstruction technique which uses the back muscle flap to form a breast with a woman's own tissue after mastectomy.

lifetime cumulative risk: all the individual yearly risks of a woman developing breast cancer added together.

lobular carcinoma in situ: considered precancerous, this "marker" is located in the deeper areas of the breast, where milk production begins.

lump: any kind of mass.

lumpectomy: a "breast conservation" surgery option in which the lump, some surrounding normal tissue and underarm lymph nodes are removed.

lymph nodes: small glands containing white

blood cells that remove waste from body tissues and that help the body fight infection.

lymphedema: a persistent swelling in the arm caused by excess fluid that collects when the lymph nodes and vessels are removed. This condition can occur many years after surgery.

M

malignant: cancerous.

mammography: the best screening process currently available for breast cancer.

mammogram: an x-ray which pictures the tissues of the breast. Mammograms should be performed by a radiologist or x-ray technician under the supervision of a radiologist.

mastectomy (modified radical): a surgery option in which the breast and lymph nodes are completely removed.

mastectomy (simple): removal of breast tissue.

mastectomy (partial, wide excision or quadrantectomy): see **lumpectomy**.

metastasize: spread to other parts of the body.

metastatic breast cancer: cancer which originated in the breast, then spread to other sites, such as liver, bones or brain.

N

needle aspiration: a type of biopsy in which a fine, hollow needle is inserted into the lump under local anesthesia, and any fluid that is present is drawn into a syringe.

negative biopsy: no cancer cells are seen.

node-negative breast cancer: breast cancer with the absence of lymph node involvement.

O

oncologist: a doctor who manages a patient's cancer and treatment.

P

pathologist: examines the biopsied tissue under a microscope, looking for abnormalities.

pathology report: the pathologist's written record of the analysis of tissue.

phantom breast: when a woman feels as if her breast were still present after a mastectomy.

plastic surgeon: a medical doctor specially trained to do cosmetic and reconstructive surgery.

prostheses: external breast forms worn by women who have had mastectomies.

protocol: course of treatment being used.

R

radiation therapy: a treatment which kills cancer cells only in the treated area.

radiation therapist: a certified technician with special training in radiation therapy.

radiation oncologist: a medical doctor who specializes in radiation therapy.

radiologist: a medical doctor who specializes in the interpretation of x-rays for diagnosis.

Reach to Recovery: a national program sponsored by the American Cancer Society, in which women who have had breast cancer visit and counsel women after surgery.

reconstructive surgery: plastic surgery which re-creates the shape of breasts.

recurrence: when a woman's breast cancer returns. Recurrences can be local or distant. Treatment and prognosis varies.

S

S-phase: a test which determines how many cancer cells are reproducing.

saline: a sterile, salt-water solution.

silicone: a synthetic material used to encase and fill some breast implants.

spiculated: a star-shaped, suspicious mass or nodule.

stereotactic biopsy: a method of obtaining tissue which combines mammography and computer-directed needle placement to evaluate an abnormality a mammogram can see but a doctor can't feel.

T

TRAM flap: also called the "tummy tuck" reconstruction option, the TRAM flap uses tissue from the lower abdomen to reconstruct a woman's breast after mastectomy.

tamoxifen: an anti-estrogen drug which blocks action of the estrogen in cells. This drug is used in hormonal therapy and is showing promise in some prevention studies.

tissue expansion: a process preceding installation of a breast implant in which a temporary, expandable implant is placed underneath the remaining muscle and skin following a mastectomy and periodically filled with fluid to gradually stretch the skin and muscle.

toxic: poisonous

TRAM-flap procedure: reconstructive surgery which re-creates the shape of breasts using abdominal tissue.

tumor: an abnormal growth of cells or tissue. Tumors can either be benign (noncancerous) or malignant (cancerous).

two-step procedure: when biopsy and treatment are performed at different times.

U

ultrasound: a painless test which uses high-frequency sound waves to determine whether a lump is liquid or solid.

Resources

Recommended for Further Reading

GENERAL BOOKS ABOUT COPING WITH CANCER

Getting Well Again, by O. Carl Simonton, M.D., Stephanie Matthews-Simonton and James L. Creighton
Bantam Books, New York, 1992
A step-by-step, self-help guide for patients and their families in dealing with cancer. Describes imaging techniques.

The Cancer Conqueror, by Greg Anderson
Andrews & McMeel, 1990
How to deal with the diagnosis of cancer in a hopeful and faithful way. A good book to read early on.

The Triumphant Patient, by Greg Anderson
Thomas Nelson Publishers, 1992
An uplifting and encouraging look at how to become your own medical specialist and increase quality of life.

Surviving Cancer, by Danette Kaufman
Acropolis Books, Acropolis Books, Ltd., 1989
Written by a breast cancer patient but pertains to all cancers. Contains very practical tips.

Cancervive, by Susan Nessim and Judith Ellis
Houghton Mifflin, 1991
How to cope with life after cancer. Includes information on insurance and fear of recurrence. Applicable to all types of cancer.

Diagnosis Cancer, by Wendy Schlessel Harpam, M.D.
W.W. Norton and Co., New York, 1992

I Can Cope, by Judi Johnson, R.N., and Linda Klein
DCI Publishing, 1988
Written by an oncology nurse, this easy-to-read book is designed to help the reader develop coping skills. A must-read for anyone diagnosed with cancer, and their families.

You Can't Afford the Luxury of Negative Thought, by John Roger and Peter McWilliams
Prelude Press, 1988
Easy to read and uplifting on how to live and die. Guilt-free reading which is humorous at times.

The American Cancer Society offers a variety of free booklets on topics relating to cancer, breast cancer, coping, diagnosis, treatment and more. For a complete list of what is available, call your local chapter.

The National Cancer Institute (NCI) also offers free cancer information. Call 301-496-5583.

GENERAL BOOKS ABOUT BREAST CANCER

Breast Cancer: The Complete Guide, by Yashaw Hirshaut, M.D., F.A.C.P. and Peter I Pressman, M.D., F.A.C.S.

Bantam Books, 1992

Thorough treatment of the subject by two physicians in private practice in New York.

The Breast Cancer Companion, by Kathy LaTour

William Morrow and Company, New York, 1993

A breast cancer survivor combines personal stories and medical information.

The Breast Cancer Handbook, by Joan Swirsky and Barbara Balaban.

Harper Collins, New York, 1994

A step-by-step guide for the woman facing biopsy and diagnosis by a clinical nurse specialist and social worker experienced in breast cancer support groups.

Confronting Breast Cancer, by Sigmund Weitzmann, M.D., Irene Kutzer, M.D., D. Phil and H.E. Pizer, PA-C

Vintage Books, 1986

Basic information about the breast, surgery, coping, nutrition and proper therapies.

Dr. Susan Love's Breast Book, by Susan Love, M.D., with Karen Lindsey

Addison-Wesley Publishing Co., Inc. 1990

Information about breast diseases and breast health, written by a national expert. A must-read for every woman, whether or not she has breast cancer.

Estrogen and Breast Cancer: A Warning to Women, by Carol Rinzler

MacMillan, 1993

This book traces the history of estrogen, linking its use to increasing breast cancer incidence.

Women's Cancers: How to Prevent Them, How to Treat Them, How to Beat Them, by Kerry McGinn and Pamela Haylock

Hunter House, 1993

A nurse and breast cancer survivor teams with a nurse and cancer-care consultant to examine the fears, myths and truths about pelvic, breast, uterine, ovarian and rare gynecologic cancers.

MASTECTOMY AND RECONSTRUCTION

Healing, A Woman's Guide to Recovery After Mastectomy, by Rosalind Delores Benedet, N.P., M.S.N.

R. Benedet Publishing, 1993

Written by a nurse practitioner, this is a short and very practical book about mastectomy and recovery, which also includes information about breast forms and exercises.

A Woman's Decision: Breast Care, Treatment and Reconstruction, by Karen Berger and John Bostwick III, M.D.

Quality Medical Publishing, Inc.

Includes a section on breast augmentation and photographs of breast treatment options.

CHEMOTHERAPY

Coping with Chemotherapy, by Nancy Bruning

Balantine, 1992

An excellent reference book which includes the author's personal experience and commentary from health professionals.

Everyone's Guide to Cancer Therapy, by Malin Dollinger, M.D., Ernest Rosenbaum, M.D., and Greg Cable

Somerville House Books, Ltd., 1991

Good, basic information on cancer and therapy. Includes information on chemotherapy, bone marrow transplants, coping and home-care resources.

COPING WITH BREAST CANCER

Affirmations, Meditations and Encouragements for Women Living with Breast Cancer, by Linda Dackman

Harper, 1991

Topics span the emotional spectrum of breast cancer diagnosis, treatment and recovery. Included are fear of recurrence, anger and living in the present. This valuable companion makes an excellent gift.

Coping When a Parent Has Cancer, by Linda L. Strauss

The Rosen Publishing Group, Inc., 1988

Aimed at teen-agers, this books provides complete and frank help for teens to continue with their lives despite a seriously ill parent.

The Healing Path, A Soul Approach to Illness, by Marc Ian Barasch

G.P. Putnam's Sons, New York, 1993

Re-frames the notion of healing to encompass more than just the physical.

How To Reduce Your Risk of Breast Cancer, by Jon J. Michnovicz, M.D., Ph.D.

Warner Books, 1994

Nutrition information and guidelines.

Now That I Have Cancer I Am Whole, by John Robert McFarland

Andrews and McMeel, Kansas City, 1993

A colon cancer patient re-examines life with humor and finds it enhanced.

Recovering From Breast Cancer, by Carol Fabian, M.D., and Andrea Warren, M.A., M.S.

Harper, 1992

Brief yet thorough treatment of basic facts about cancer through coping and recovery. Short resource list, no photos.

Spinning Straw Into Gold, by Ronnie Kaye

S & S Trade, 1991

A counselor shares her own experience with breast cancer and a recurrence with wit and understanding. Also included are suggestions for coping and full emotional recovery from breast cancer. Excellent section for single women.

Surviving A Writer's Life, by Suzanne Lipsett

Harper, San Francisco

Insights about breast cancer, mastectomy, recovery, recurrence and the fear and pain with which all women must cope.

Women Talk About Breast Surgery, From Diagnosis to Recovery, by Amy Gross and Dee Ito

Clarkson Potter Publishers, 1990

A book of personal vignettes which touches on insurance and patient rights. Not all positive.

PERSONAL STORIES

Breast Cancer Journal: A Century of Petals, by Juliet Wittman

Fulcrum Publications, 1993

This journalist, actress and feminist shares her personal experience with breast cancer.

Cancer As A Woman's Issue, by Midge Stocker, Ed.

Third Side Press, 1988

Essays on breast cancer from a variety of perspectives, including women of all ages, and exploration of lesbian issues.

Getting Better, by Ann A. Hargrove, Ph.D.

CompCare Publishers, 1988

A memorable, sometimes humorous account of the author's breast cancer experience as a single mother.

No Less A Woman: Ten Women Shatter the Myths About Breast Cancer, by Deborah H. Kahane, M.S.W.

S & S Trade, 1993

A historical and cultural perspective on breast cancer.

My Breast, by Joyce Wadler

Pocket Books, 1992

Humorous story of the author's encounter with breast cancer and the man who wasn't there for her.

One in Three: Women With Cancer Confront an Epidemic, edited by Judy Brady

Cleis Press, 1991

Personal stories of 41 women. Also included is a backdrop of socioeconomic history and a lesson in the ins and outs of the cancer establishment.

RISK

Relative Risk: Living with a Family History of Breast Cancer, by N.C. Baker

Viking Press, 1991

Information for the woman who fears her risk of developing breast cancer, complete with data that puts the risk into perspective.

If It Runs In Your Family, by M.D. Eades

New York, 1991

RECONSTRUCTION

Breast Implants: Everything You Need to Know, by Nancy Bruning

Hunter House, 1992

A look at the latest information from consumer health advocates, the Federal Drug Administration and the medical community.

Saline Implant Clinical Trials
Food & Drug Administration
1-800-532-4440

Breast Implants Hotline
1-800-892-9211

SIGNIFICANT OTHERS & SEXUALITY

Man To Man: When the Woman You Love Has Breast Cancer, by Andy Murcia and Bob Stewart
St. Martin's Press, New York, 1989
A helpful account of the authors' reactions to their wives' breast cancer battles, by the husband of movie star Ann Jillian and a friend. Includes helpful suggestions for significant others.

Intimacy: Living As a Woman After Cancer, by Jacquelyn Johnson
NC Press Ltd., Toronto, 1987
Frank treatment of issues of sexuality after all types of cancer. Extensive bibliography and resource list included.

CHILDREN'S BOOKS

When Eric's Mom Fought Cancer, by Judith Vigna
Albert Whitman & Company, 1993

NEWSLETTERS

National Alliance of Breast Cancer Organizations (NABCO)
1180 Avenue of the Americas, second floor
New York, NY 10036

The National Women's Health Network
(Women's Health Information Service)
1325 G Street, NW
Washington, D.C. 20005

Breast Cancer Action
55 New Montgomery St.
San Francisco, CA 94105
415-243-9301
415-243-3996 (fax)

OTHER RESOURCES
American Cancer Society
1599 Clifton Road, N.E.
Atlanta, Ga., 30329
1-800-ACS-2345

National Cancer Institute
1-800-4-CANCER

National Alliance of Breast Cancer Organizations (NABCO)
Second floor, 1180 Avenue of the Americas
New York, NY 10036
212-719-0154

Nolvadex (Tamoxifen) Patient Assistance Program
1-800-424-3727

Susan G. Komen Foundation
Dallas, TX
1-800-462-9273 (Helpline)
214-450-1777

Y-ME National Breast Cancer Organization
1-800-221-2141
312-986-8228 (24-hour hotline)
http://www.y-me.org

RESOURCES ON THE INTERNET
Allexperts.com is a site where breast cancer survivors answer questions
http://www.allexperts.com/getExpert.asp?category=1001

AMC Cancer Research Center researches the causes of breast cancer
http://www.amc.org/

Blood & Bone Marrow Transplant Newsletter is a non-profit organization that provides informal to bone marrow, peripheral blood stem cell and cord blood transplant patients.
http://www.bmtnews.org/

The Breast Cancer Book Store is, in association with Amazon.com, the Internet's largest online bookseller.
http://members.aol.com/healthbook/breastcancer/index.htm

Cancer Information Service is a National Instutudes of Health site
http://cancernet.nci.nih.gov/clinpdq/soa/Breast cancer Physician.html

Celebrating Life Foundation is one of the leading foundations that promote breast cancer awareness which specifically targets women of color.
http://www.celebratinglife.org/

Index

About the Authors

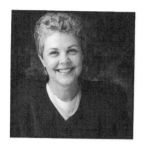

Suzanne W. Braddock, M.D., a breast cancer survivor, is a dermatologist in private practice in Omaha, Neb. Born and raised in New Jersey, Dr. Braddock received her medical training at the Medical College of Pennsylvania, Philadelphia, and at the University of Nebraska School of Medicine, Omaha. Dr. Braddock is the author of several scientific publications.

Her daughter, Gail, has been a friend and source of joy throughout her diagnosis and recovery.

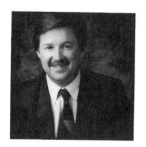

John Edney, M.D., F.A.C.S., a plastic surgeon in private practice in Omaha, Neb., specializes in post-mastectomy breast reconstruction and cosmetic surgery. Dr. Edney is an assistant clinical professor of surgery at the University of Nebraska School of Medicine, Omaha. He attended Creighton University School of Medicine. Dr. Edney and his wife, Pat, have three children, Christopher, Matthew and Jennifer.

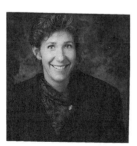

Jane Kercher, M.D., F.A.C.S., is a general and oncological surgeon in Denver, Colorado. She received her medical training at the University of Utah Medical School in Salt Lake City, Utah, and at the University of Nebraska. She has been an assistant professor at the University of Nebraska School of Medicine, Department of Surgery.

A native of Wyoming, Dr. Kercher now lives in Denver with her son, Matthew.

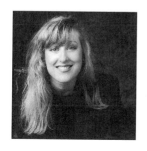

Melanie Morrissey Clark has a B.S. in Journalism from the University of Nebraska at Omaha in Omaha, Neb. She is the editor of *Today's Omaha Woman* magazine and co-owner of Clark Creative Group.

Melanie lives in Omaha with her husband, Fred, and children Cooper, Sophie and Simon.

Addicus Books

Visit the Addicus Books Web Site:
www.AddicusBooks.com

Straight Talk About Breast Cancer $12.95
    Suzanne Braddock, MD / 1-886039-21-6

Overcoming Postpartum Depression and Anxiety $12.95
    Linda Sebastian, RN, MN, ARNP / 1-886930-34-8

The Stroke Recovery Book $14.95
    Kip Burkman, MD / 1-886039-30-5

The Healing Touch—Keeping the Doctor/Patient $9.95
    Relationship Alive Under Managed Care
    David Cram, MD / 1-886039-31-3

Hello, Methuselah! Living to 100 and Beyond $14.95
    George Webster, PhD / 1-886039-25-9

The Family Compatibility Test $9.95
    Susan Adams / 1-886039-27-5

First Impressions—Tips to Enhance Your Image $14.95
    Joni Craighead / 1-886039-26-7

Prescription Drug Abuse—The Hidden Epidemic $14.95
    Rod Colvin / 1-886039-22-4

Please send:

_____ copies of_____

at $ _____ each   TOTAL   _____

Nebr. residents add 6.5% sales tax   _____
Shipping/Handling
$3.20 for first book.
$1.10 for each additional book.   _____

                    TOTAL ENCLOSED   _____

Name _____

Address _____

City _____ State _____ Zip _____

☐ Visa   ☐ Master Card   ☐ Am. Express

Credit card number _____ Exp. date _____

Order by credit card, personal check or money order.
Send to:

Addicus Books
Mail Order Dept.
P.O. Box 45327
Omaha, NE 68145
Or, order TOLL FREE: 800-352-2873
or online at: www.AddicusBooks.com